Dr. Armin Fischer

Female Pelvic Floor Disorders and their Successful Conservative Treatment

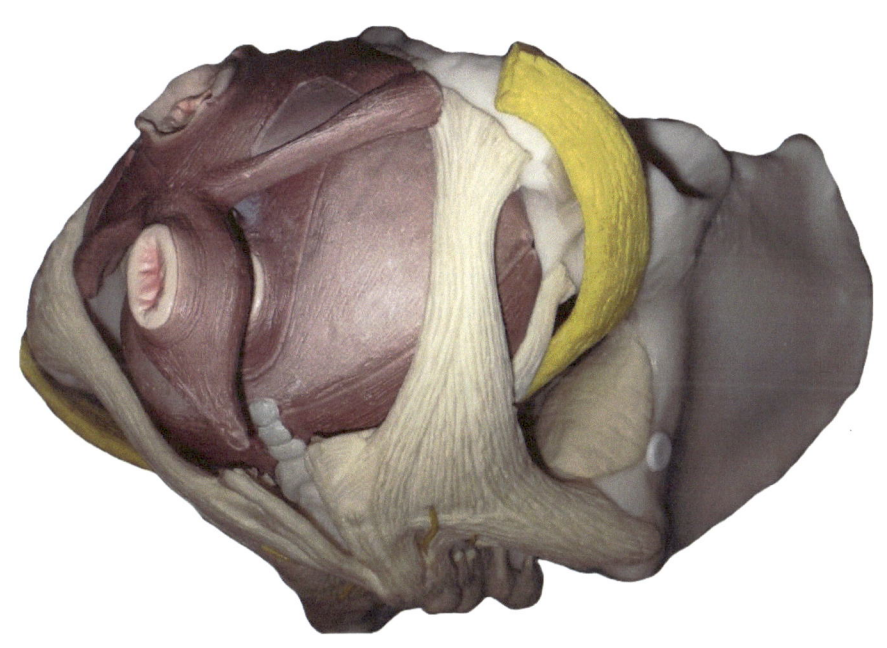

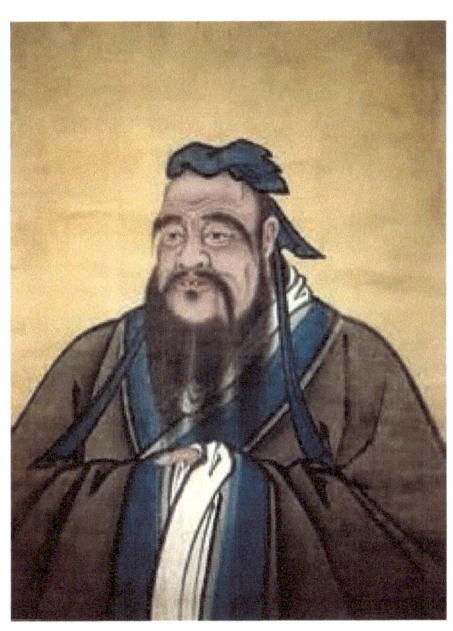

By three methods we may learn wisdom:
First, by reflection, which is noblest;
Second, by imitation, which is easiest;
and third by experience, which is the bitterest.

                                      Confucius

Foreword

Female pelvic floor disorders are a very common disease. Many women suffer in silence and dare not speak about it to their closest and/or the doctor. Watching TV one gets the impression that panty liners, pads and diapers should lead to a sufficient life quality and that incontinence treated that was is not a big problem. There is no sufficient information publically available on female genital descent, its interaction with continence and surgery at the moment seems to be the only treatment available. Using minimally invasive procedures for prolapse surgery and tapes for incontinence surgery surgeons promise only a little discomfort and pain after surgery, good and long lasting results often neglecting to talk about risk, side-effects, and implications on further every day life or behavior.

The number of women affected is much higher than the number seeking treatment, the number of women undergoing surgery without previous conservative treatment much too high. Conservative treatment not only helps to diminish the number of operations needed, but also helps to improve postoperative long-term results of surgical interventions and is a good means to delay surgery. One might ask why the delay of surgery is a goal worthy to achieve. The answer to that is one of the easier ones in urogynaecology. There are only a limited number of interventions possible in one woman's lifetime, and the later surgical treatment starts the better the chances to have a symptom-free life in the old days, very important as the life-span of man extends in the average.

The focus of this booklet lies on three aspects of urogynaecological treatment
- Understanding of structure and function of the pelvic floor
- Understanding of its pathologies
- Knowledge of possible conservative treatments to prevent, precede, improve and conserve pelvic floor surgery an its results.

But the most important rue to follow is:
Do not undergo surgery before conservative treatment is completely used to its full capacity.

Chapter 1: The Pelvic Floor - structure and function

1.1 Anatomy - the basics

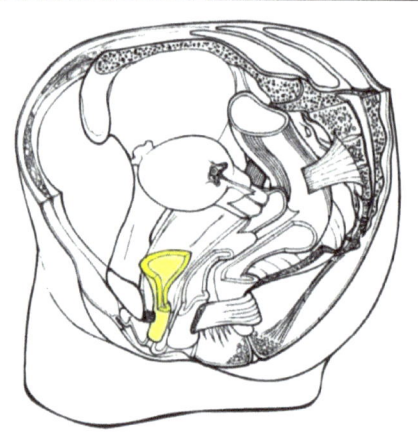

Bladder and Urethra
The bladder rests on the anterior vaginal wall, it has no fixation of its own at the pelvic wall level. The urethra on the other hand has surrounding connective tissue that connects to the pelvic bone an plays an important role in establishing female urinary continence under stress conditions (pubo-urethral ligament).

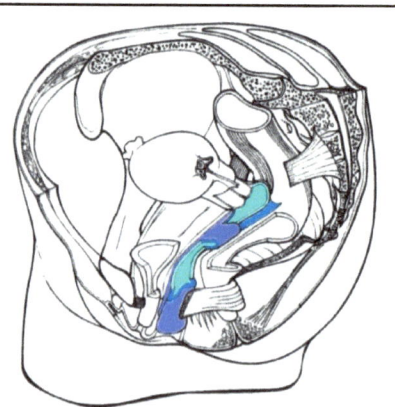

Vagina and Uterus
Those structures in the pelvic floor's center contribute largely to stability (and form) of the adjacent systems. They stabilize bladder and rectum through their connective tissues adherent to bones and muscles in their vicinity. The cervix resembles functionally the center stone of a dome and is hence only expendable when good reasons ask for its removal (bad Pap smear, HPV-infection,...)

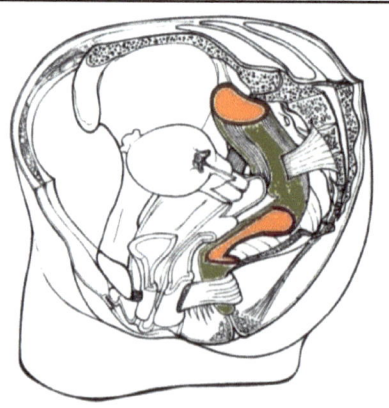

Sigma, Rectum and Anus
The anus with its inner and outer sphincter system and the mucosa of the anoderm connected to the lower rectum are very susceptible to childbirth-related trauma and suffer defect due to tears and cuts that lead to defects in the endopelvic fascia. Those may have bad influence on defecation und anal continence.

Fig. 1: The three compartments of the pelvic floor system

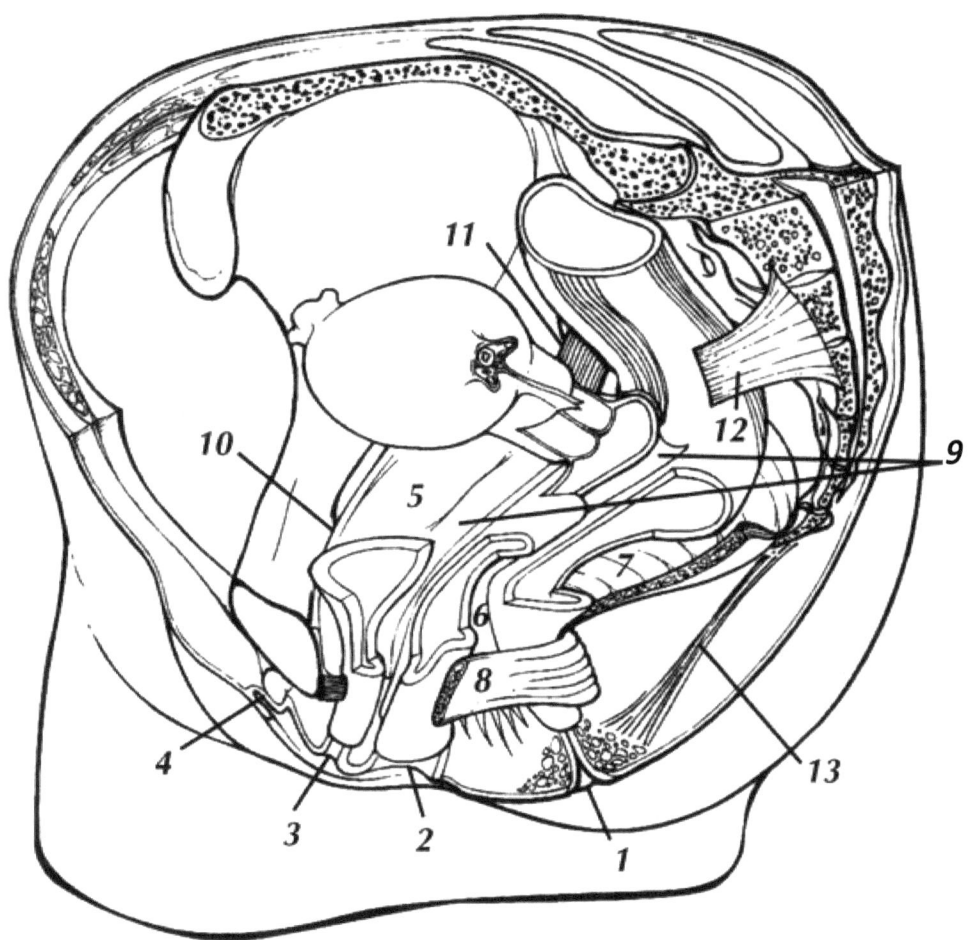

Fig. 2: The anatomic structures of the pelvic floor system

1	=	Anus
2	=	Vagina
3	=	Meatus urethrae externus **(external orifice of the urethra)**
4	=	Clitoris
5	=	Lamina pubocervicalis fasciae endopelvinae
6	=	Lamina rectovaginalis fasciae endopelvinae
7	=	M. levator ani **(Levator ani muscle)**
8	=	M. puborectalis (Pars puborectalis m. lev. ani)
9	=	endopelvic fascia
10	=	Arcus tendineus fasciae endopelvinae
11	=	Spina ischiadica **(ischiadic spine)**
12	=	Lig. sacrouterinum **(uterosacral ligament)**
13	=	Lig. anococcygeum

The endopelvic fascia is trapezoid-shaped and located slightly above the plane of the levator ani muscles leaving an aperture for the rectum and for childbirth. Of great importance is the connection of the endopelvic fascia to the arcus tendineous of the pelvic floor muscles (insertion of intern obturator muscle to levator ani muscle) the socalled whiteline. Weakness or tears at this level lead to important dysfunction of the pelvic floor system as will be shown later.

Fig. 3: anatomy of the endopelvic fascia

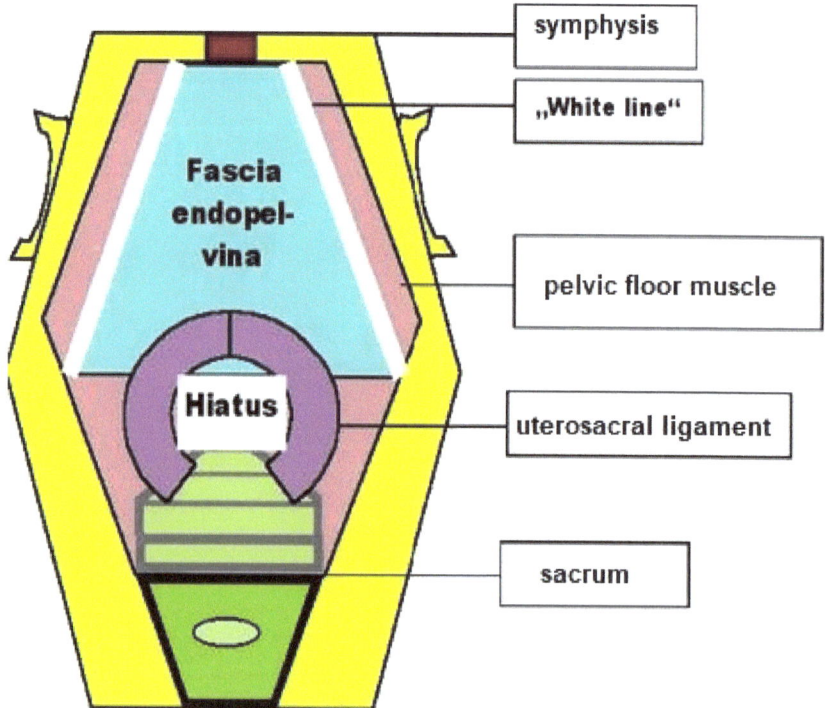

The vagina incorporated into the endopelvic fascia layer is devided into two segments: the lower thrid following the inclination of the urethra, the upper two thirds forming a 130 angle to the lower third are connected to the endopelvic fascia on both sides forming the lateral sulcus anteriolerly and to the rectovaginal sheath of the endopelvic fascia on its posterior wall.

Fig.4: threedimensional anatomy of the vagina

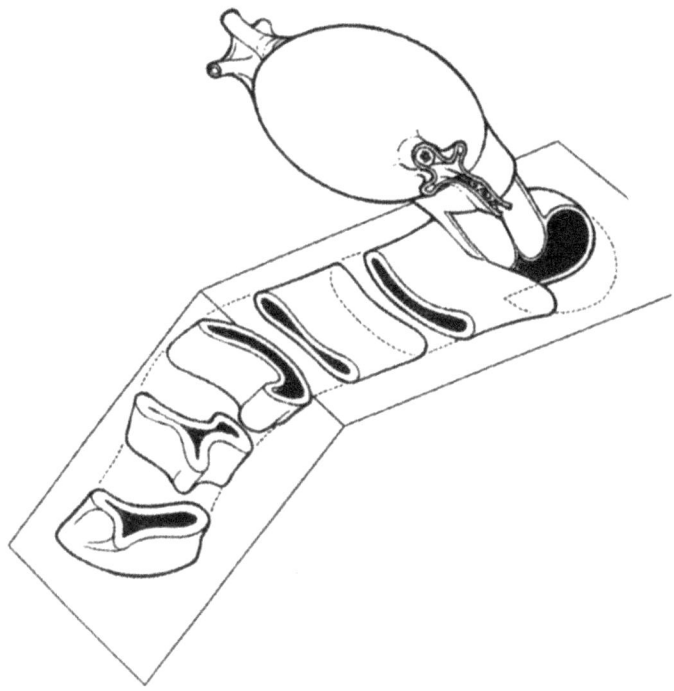

1.2 Continence and Integral Theory

Up to the late 1990's (ntroduction of TVT surgical procedure) the explanation of continence was mainly based on two theoretical concepts
ENHORNING's pressure equalisation theory of the 60's and DeLANCEY's hammock theory of the early 90's.

Raised intraabdominal pressure closes off the urethra provided the proximal urethra is correctly positioned in the pressure sphere of the abdominal cavity (Enhörning, 1961). 30 years later DeLancey (1991) came up with the hammock theory ruling out that the loss of the suburethral support by the underlying vagina leads to a loss of stress continence.

The rise of pressure inside the urethra during effort greatly exceeds the rise immediately outside the urethra, the critical factor for stress continence being the tightness of the vaginal hammock.

In 1993 British scientists came up with the disturbing finding, that the incidence of detrusor instability being up to 18% after bladder neck suspension. As a consequence patients with instable detrusor were not to be recommended to undergo surgery. As vaginal stretching and elevating towards the pubic bone exert chronic pressure on the bladder base nerve endings from behind causing their premature activation: nocturia, frequency and urge arise. Interpreting detrusor instability as a prematurely activated otherwise normal micturition reflex by distortion of the underlying vaginal wall and its reversal with digital support of the bladder base area of the vagina in cases without significant bladder neck elevation sheds a quite different light on the surgical curability of states of instable detrusor.

Petros and Ulmsten published their so called Integral Theory also in 1991. This being of enormous complexity and based on the assumption that female urinary tract disorders are based on connective tissue dysfunction it lasted over half a decade until with the introduction of TVT a larger number of doctors got acquainted with their ideas and most likely the majority of even frequent users of TVT still do not fully comprehend the theoretical concept behind the method.

1.2.1 Continence and Bladder Function according to the Integral Theory

Bladder dysfunction is secondary to anatomical dysfunction. The theory states that both urinary dysfunction and vaginal prolapse have a common origin, i.e., laxity in the vagina or its supporting ligaments/structures.

A classification of laxity in 3 zones of the vagina guides both surgical treatment and new pelvic floor rehabilitation methods.

The aim of therapy is the reestablishment of a balance of (muscle) forces that enables closing and opening of the bladder neck for voiding and keeping the detrusor at rest during filling of the bladder (Figure 5 – Petros' Trampoline Analogy).

Fig. 5: Petros' Trampoline Analogy

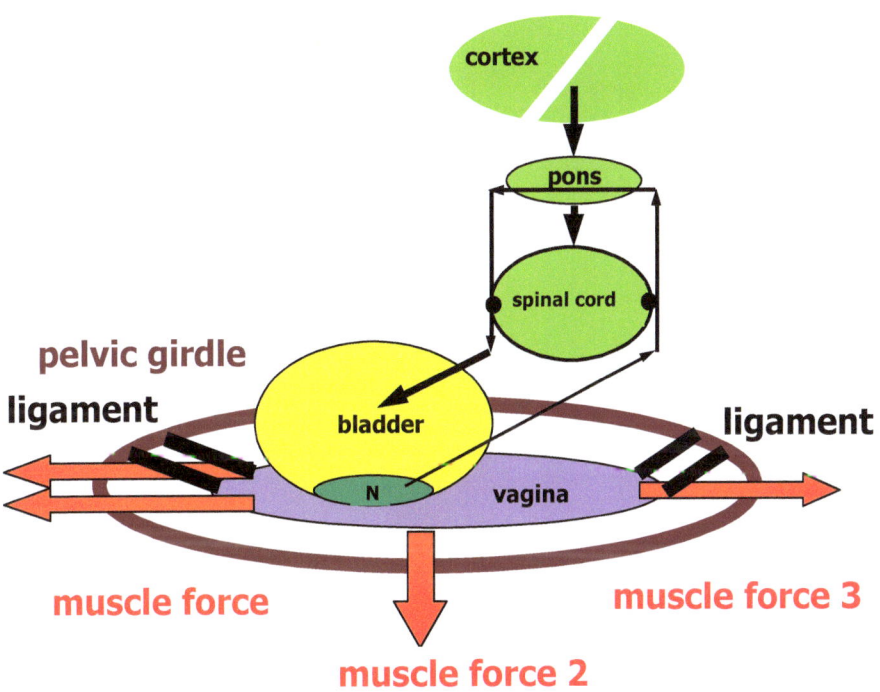

Using analogies the understanding of the theory may be facilitated. For example: compare the pelvic system to a bridge suspended over a large river. You can find some analogies:

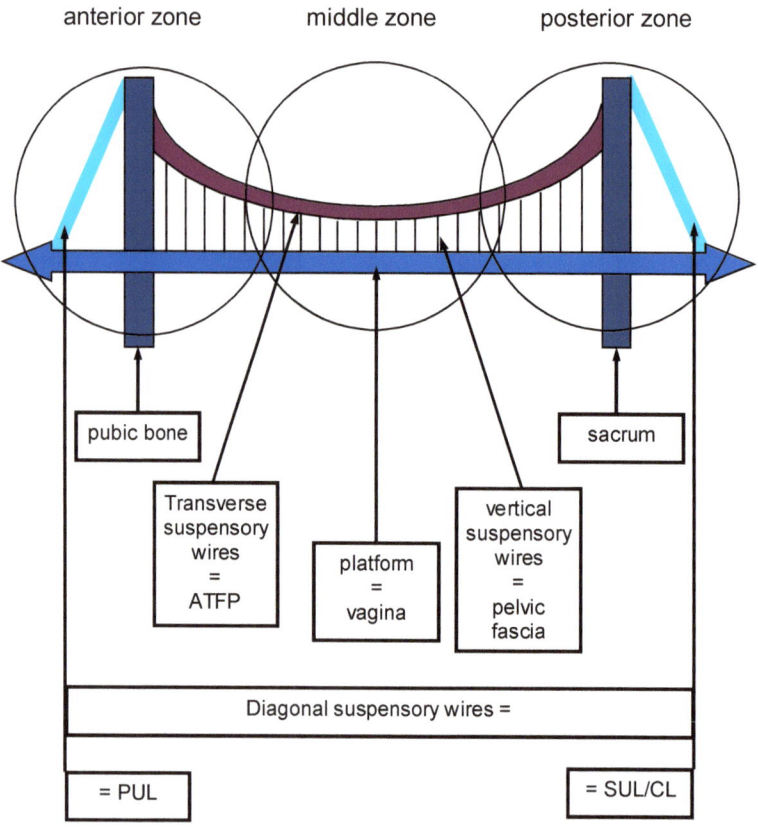

Fig. 6: Bridge Analogy
ATFP: arcus tendineous of endopelvic fascia
PUL: pubourthral ligament
SUL: utrosacral ligament
CL: cardinal ligament

Now the anatomy has to simplified in an appropriate way to match the way pelvic floor function is described in the Integral Theory. The main elements have to be represented:

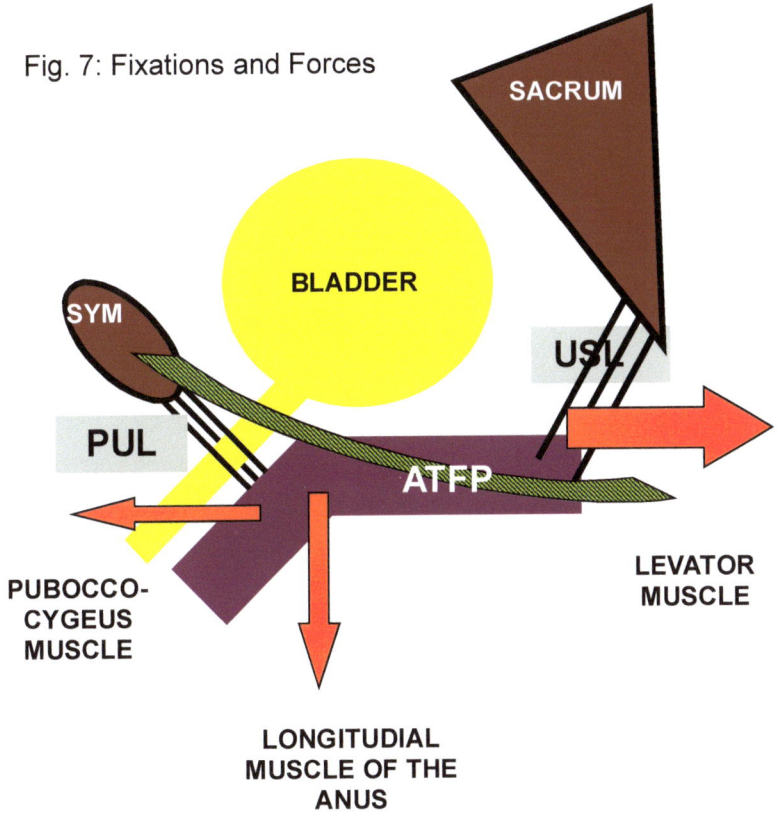

Fig. 7: Fixations and Forces

The comprehension of the Integral Theory (even of it's simplified version) is essential for the understanding of bladder function and its disorders.

-the striated muscles of the pelvic floor stretch the collagen of the pelvic organs to achieve their shape and function
-pubourethral ligament in front, the arcus tendineous fasciae pelvis in the middle on both sides, the cardinal ligament in the middle to both sides and the uterosacral ligament to the back anchor the organs and transmit the forces, their elastic component serving as a "shock absorber" and energy storing facility for the restoration of the organ's initial shape

-3 muscle forces act on the pelvic structures to bring them to function
- backward force stretches upper vagina/bladder base backwards during stress
- forward forces stretch the hammock forwards to close urethra from behind
- downward force rotates the upper vagina around the pubourethral ligment

-PUL transmits backward and forward forces to the pubic symphysis
-ATFP assists in the transmission of backward forces to PUL
-USL transmits downward forces to coccyx and sacrum

therefore:
relaxation of the forward forces allow the backward forces to open the outflow tract.
Contraction of the forward forces close off the outflow tract.

A ship's sail (vagina) is useless unless it is tightened against the mast and ship (bones) by its ropes (ligaments) to transmit the wind's force (muscle contraction) sufficiently to drive the boat forward (urethral closure).

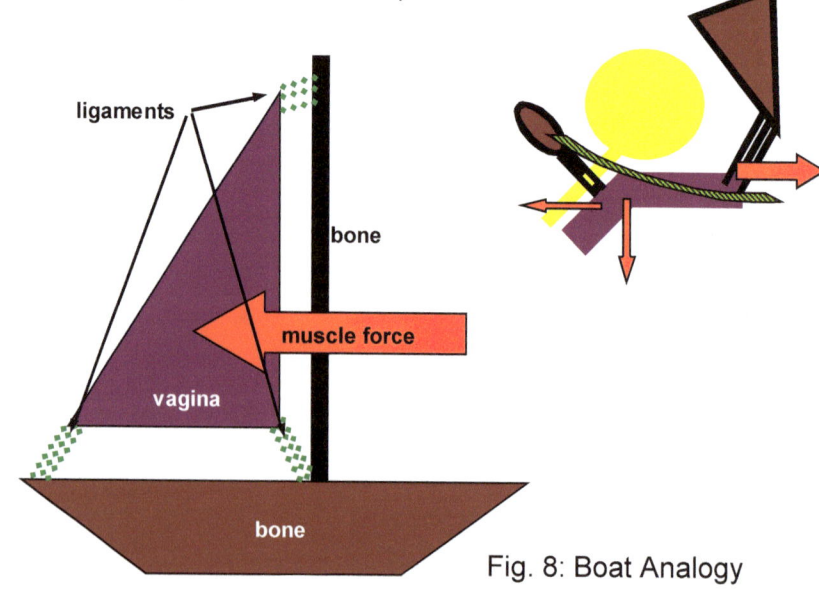

Fig. 8: Boat Analogy

Dysfunction may be for one thing the result of vaginal (hammock) or suspensory ligament laxity dissipating the forces which stretch the vagina to close the outflow tract.

Mid-urethral support is needed to cure stress incontinence by
-tightening the hammock and
-restoring the pubourethral ligaments as insertion points for the forward
 and backward forces
The role of the posterior fixation of the vagina (USL) is to provide the necessary downward forces to enable the upper vaginal rotation around PUL.

Laxity of anterior and posterior ligaments prevent the vagina from stretching during bladder filling to support the bladder's hydrostatic pressure. This stimulates the stretch receptors at the bladder base.
A lax vagina cannot be stretched. The receptors fire off at a lower volume causing the premature activation of a normal micturition reflex. Patients suffer from bladder instability symptoms such as nocturia, frequency or urgency.

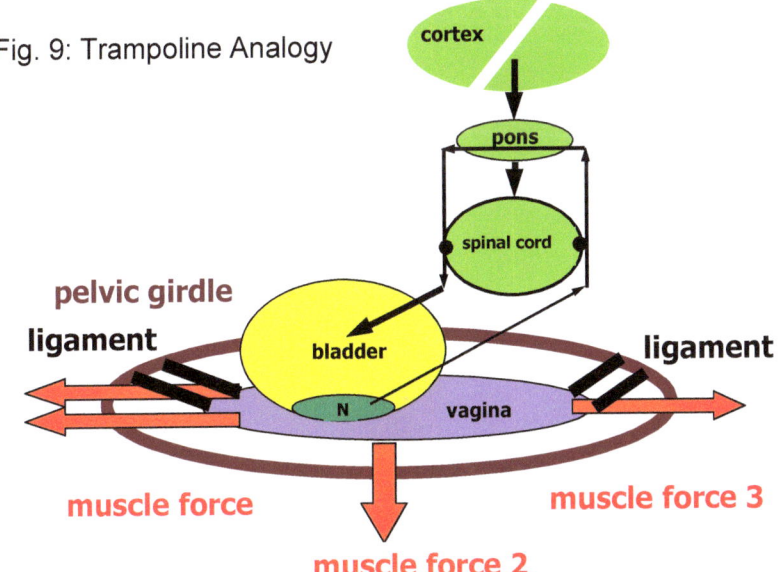

Fig. 9: Trampoline Analogy

Closure is obtained by 3 different movements:
1. 1st movement: backward force stretches rectum, ATFP und upper vagina backwards against PUL (pre-tensioning of the hammock)
2. 2nd movement: forward force pulls hammock forward
3. 3rd movement: downward force pulls rectum and upper vagina downwards against USL and CL

Both vagina and urethra/bladder base are attached to one another by fibroligamentous structures only in the area of the distal urethra/lower vagina and the bladder base/upper vagina. The proximal urethra remains unattached.

Inherent vaginal elasticity and slow-twitch muscle contraction maintain urethral closure at rest. Active closure in coughing or staining is achieved by activating the backward forces to pull bladder neck, upper vagina and rectum downward and backward by angulation of the superior border of the levator muscle and the forward forces to pull ascending vagina and urethra forwards creating a right-angled bend in the urethra on both sides of the insertion of PUL. Relaxation of PCM (or laxity of the ligaments) induce micturition by funnelling inducing the micturition reflex.

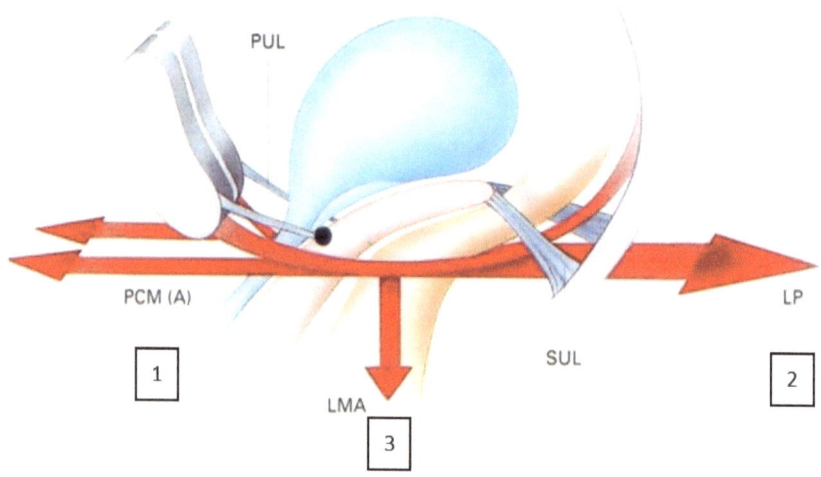

Fig. 10: Three different movements

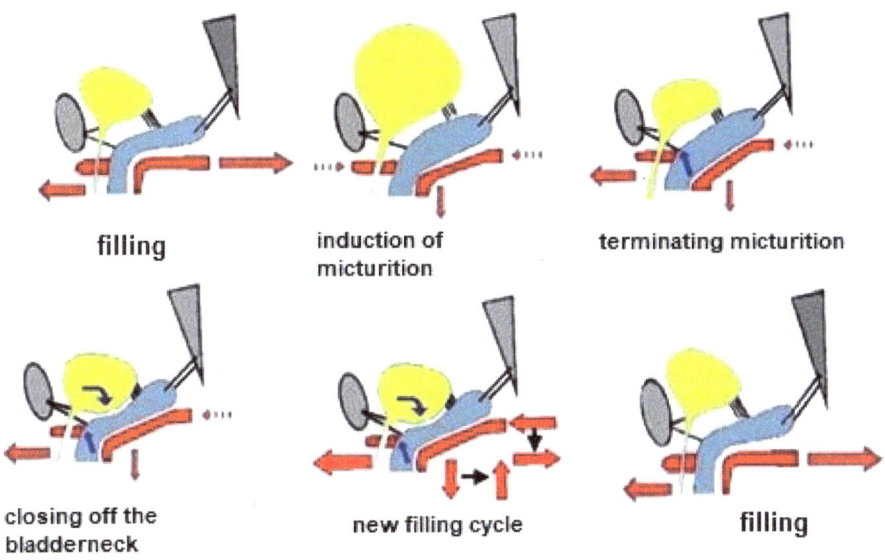

Fig. 11: Micturition cycle

PCM(A): anteriorer part of pubococcygeus mucle
LP: Levatorplate
LMA: longitudinal muscle to the anus

Table 1: Interaction of structures during the bladder cycle

	PCM(A)	subure-thral vagina	bladder neck	detrusor muscle	LP	LMA
filling	C	moves towards symphysis	closed	R	C	R
Induction of voiding	R	reduced tension	open	C	R	C
micturition	R	funneling	open	C	R	C
closing off	C	C	closed	R	R	C
filling	C	moves towards symphysis	closed	R	C	R

Table 2: Imbalance occurs through strengthening/ weakening of the following structures/states

Anterior compartment	Posterior compartment
Pubourethral ligament	Levator-Plate
Burch-Colposuspension-Sutures	Longitudinal muscle to the anus
Scars after colporrhaphy or (fascia)l slings	Uterosacral ligaments
Degeneration of collagen and connective tissues	Surgery (sacrospinous fixation, sacropexy)

Bladder neck opening and closure are a function of the regular equilibrium between the muscle groups acting on the bladder neck. A disorder in equilibrium produces a functional impairment. If these functions are compared with those of a scales, an increase in the forces acting towards the front induces (e.g. by introduction of a tape replacing the defective pubourethral ligament) also an imbalance just like the weakening of the forces directed towards the back, which are responsible for the opening of the bladder neck (Tab. 1).

Urgency develops through early/premature stimulation of the pressoreceptors (green) in the bladder neck area. This stimulation, which is also associated with an imbalance, is in turn closely related to the suburethral vaginal anatomy. Relaxation and tension of the suburethral vagina (violet) produce this functional disorder due to a deficient action of these tension-producing forces (grey arrows) of a reflex-controlled contraction of the pubococcygeus muscle (grey bars). This fails to relieve the receptor-carrying area, the stimulation of the receptors (blue star) triggers urgency and/or produces a premature micturition reflex (Fig. 14, cf. also Fig.16).

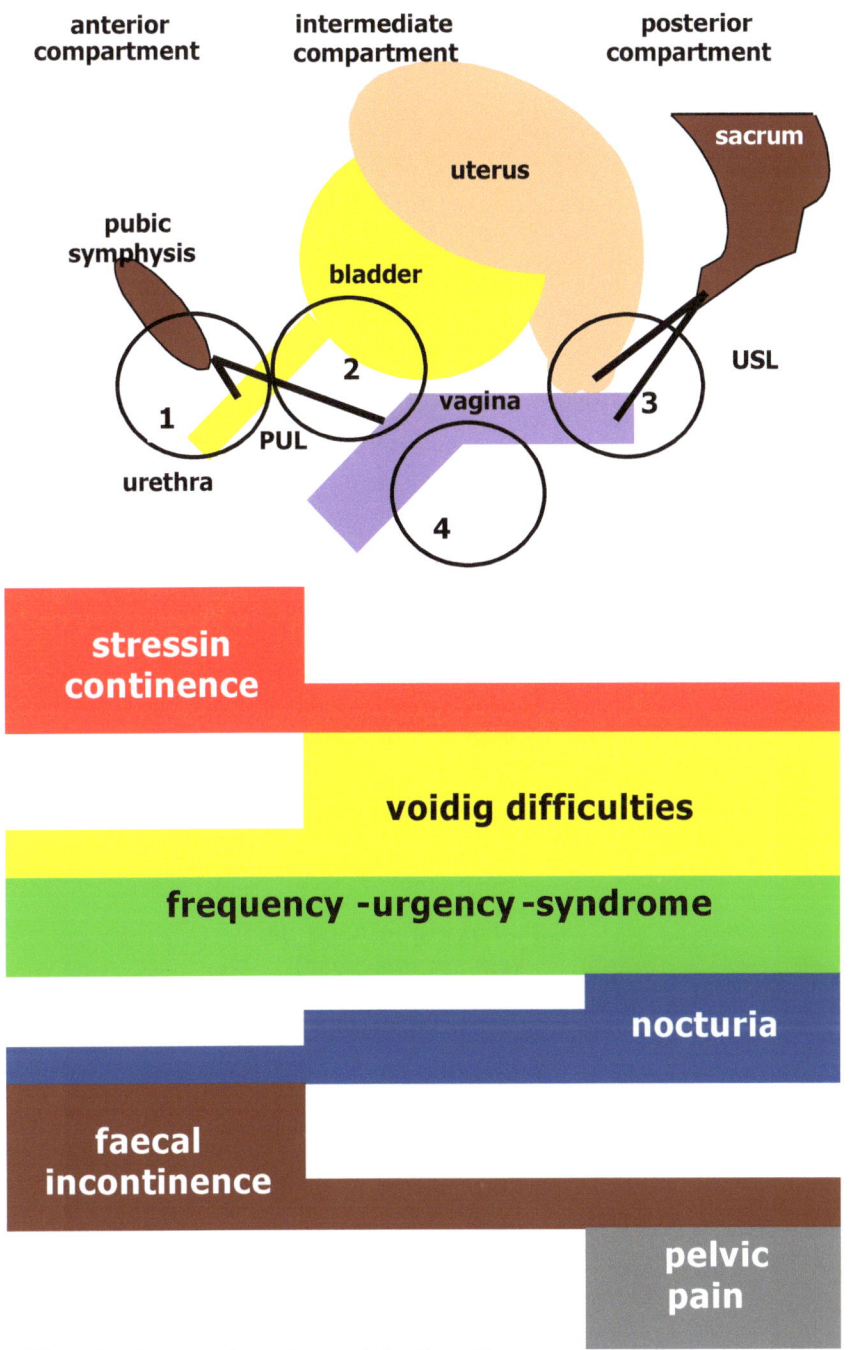

Fig. 12: Compartments and dysfunction

1.3 Diagnostic Algorithm

Anterior defect (excess laxity)	Middle defect (excess laxitiy)	Posterior defect (excess laxitiy)
Principal symptoms	**Principal symptoms**	**Principal symptoms**
Severe SI	Voiding difficulties	Incontinence worse 1 week before period
Urine loss on standing	FI persisting after post IVS	Pain (low abdomen, low sacral, dyspareunia)
Post-stress instability "always damp"		Voiding difficulties
	Principal signs	Nocturia
Faecal incontinence (FI)	Cystocele	
Nocturnal enuresis cured at puberty or wet since childhood	ATFP defect	
Principal signs	**Urodynamics**	**Principal signs**
Lax hammock	Raised rsidual	Excitation pain (vaginal and cervical)
Positive pad test (SI)	Slow emptying time	Prolapse (uterus, enterocele)
Positive midurethral Boney Funnelling on PNS	Positive PTR (Valsalva) with SI	
		Urodynamics

Tethered vagina syndrome (excess tightness)

uncommon (5%)
iatrogenic
may occur years after vaginal surgery/BNS
"motor"-DI getting out of bed
often no major SI
UVJ prolapse at strain

Tethered vagina syndrome (excess tightness)
- uncommon (5%)
- **iatrogenic**
- may occur years after vaginal surgery/BNS
- "motor"-DI getting out of bed
- often no major SI

Urodynamics
Positive CTR with SI
Stress related DI

Raised residual
Slow emptying time
Positive PTR (Valsalva) with SI

note:
FNU (frequency, nocturia and urgency may occur with all defects)
Not all criteria may be present in a particular defect

Table 3a: Diagnostic Algorithm I

Anterior defect (excess laxity)	Middle defect (excess laxity)	Posterior defect (excess laxity)
Principal symptoms	Principal symptoms	Principal symptoms
Severe SI = 90%	Voiding difficulties = 50%	Incontinence worse 1 week before period = 80%
Urine loss on standing = 90%	FI persisting after post IVS	Pain (low abdomen = 90%, low sacral = 50%, dyspareunia = 80%)
Post-stress instability = 80%		Voiding difficulties
"always damp" = 80%	Principal signs	Nocturia
Faecal incontinence (FI)	Cystocele	
Nocturnal enuresis cured at puberty or wet since childhood = 90%	ATFP defect	
Principal signs	Urodynamics	Principal signs
Lax hammock	Raised residual = 50%	Excitation pain (vaginal and cervical)
Positive pad test (SI) = 90%	Slow emptying time	Prolapse (uterus, enterocele)
Positive midurethral Boney = 95%	Positive PTR (Valsalva) with SI	

Tethered vagina syndrome (excess tightness)		
uncommon (5%)		
iatrogenic		
may occur years after vaginal surgery/BNS		
"motor"-DI getting out of bed		
often no major SI		
Funnelling on PNS = 90%		
UVJ prolapse at strain = 70%		Urodynamics
Urodynamics		Raised residual
Positive CTR with SI		Slow emptying time
Stress related DI		Positive PTR (Valsalva) with SI

Table 3b: Diagnostic Algorithm II

1.3.1 EXPLANATION OF THE DIAGNOSTIC ALGORITHM

The anatomical defects are confirmed by vaginal examination. In many cases the diagnosis becomes pictorially evident. The **anterior zone** is distal to the transverse sulcus of bladder neck, the **midzone** between this and the cervix, and the **posterior zone** behind the cervix.
NOTE: even a 1st degree of prolapse may cause symptoms; **the amount of prolapse is not linearly related to the quantum of symptoms**.

1.3.1.1 Anterior zone defects
The three directional closure forces which mechanically close the outflow tract effectively act against the anterior ligamentous supports of the vagina. Therefore stress incontinence (genuine stress incontinence) is the main manifestation of anterior zone defect. Anything preventing watertight closure of the vaginal hammock may inactivate the forward closure force (continuous leakage, unconscious incontinence). FNU may occur because of failure of the forward forces to stretch the vagina sufficiently to support the vaginal tension at the level of insertion of the utrosacral ligaments. Faecal incontinence is included because it was cured in almost 100% of cases following posterior vaginal wall re-attachment.

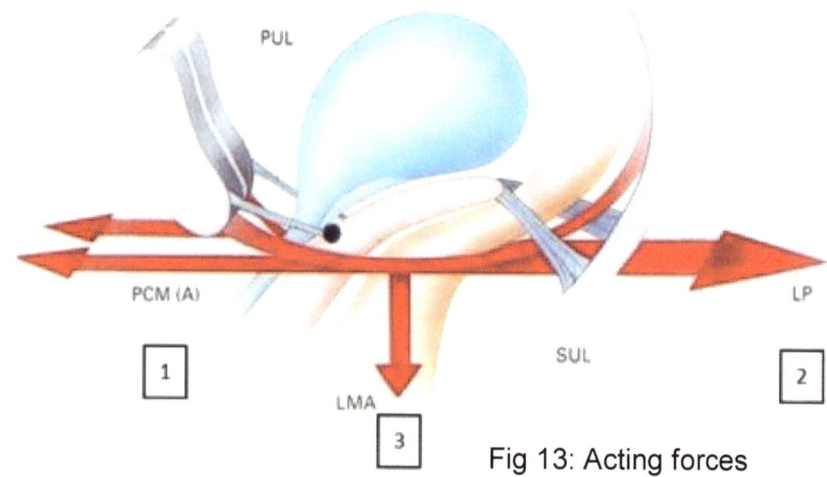

Fig 13: Acting forces

A cough transmission ratio (CTR) above 100% in the proximal urethra changing to less than 100% in the distal urethra may signify excessive stretching and narrowing of the proximal urethra by the backward forces, figure 12, induced by pubourethral ligament laxity. CTR <100% in the distal urethra may signify hammock laxity.
Midzone defects may prevent the backward and downward forces from mechanically stretching open the urethra, and may invalidate the bladder neck closure mechanism, figure 12.

Therefore emptying symptoms (underactivity, overflow incontinence, postmicturition dribble) and urodynamic indicators such as slow peak or mean flow rate, prolonged emptying time, raised residual urine etc. are also an important component of mid zone defects, figure 12. FNU may occur because of failure of the backward forces to stretch the vagina sufficiently to support the posterior part of the vagina, and stress incontinence, (albeit less frequently), because of their failure to pretension the vaginal hammock.

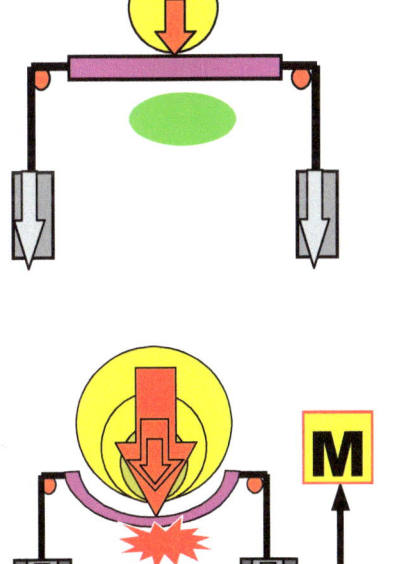

Fig. 14: tensioning of vagina and micturition reflex

Tensioning of the vagina during bladder-filling and induction of micturition – also being the mechanism for premature induction of micturition reflex in bad muscle function or loosening of the vagina

1.3.1.2 Posterior zone defects
The downward force is a key component in mechanically stretching open the bladder base during micturition, but also during closure.
Therefore emptying symptoms (underactivity, overflow incontinence, postmicturition dribble) and urodynamic indicators such as slow peak or mean flow rate, prolonged emptying time, raised residual urine etc. are an important component of posterior zone defects, figure12.
A positive Valsalva PTR in the presence of stress incontinence has been described as an important objective sign in posterior zone laxity. Restoration of the posterior ligaments, the insertion point of the downward force, frequently improves genuine stress incontinence, urge incontinence, nocturia ,detrusor instability, sensory urgency, especially in patients with prior hysterectomy. Hysterectomy would predispose to middle and posterior zone laxity. We therefore advise uterine conservation where possible. Though nocturia may occur with laxity in all 3 zones, we have found empirically that nocturia occurs more frequently with posterior zone defects, perhaps in a ratio of 4 to 1. We hypothesize that in the supine patient, lax posterior ligaments may not adequately support the distending bladder base, allowing the stretch receptors to fire off prematurely, so that the urge symptoms cause the patient to wake and go to the toilet, nocturia. This concept is better understood by rotating figure 15 clockwise at 90 degrees. Non-urinary symptoms caused by vaginal laxity confer greater accuracy upon the algorithm. Pelvic pain of otherwise unknown origin has been cured by repairing laxity in the posterior ligaments of vagina.

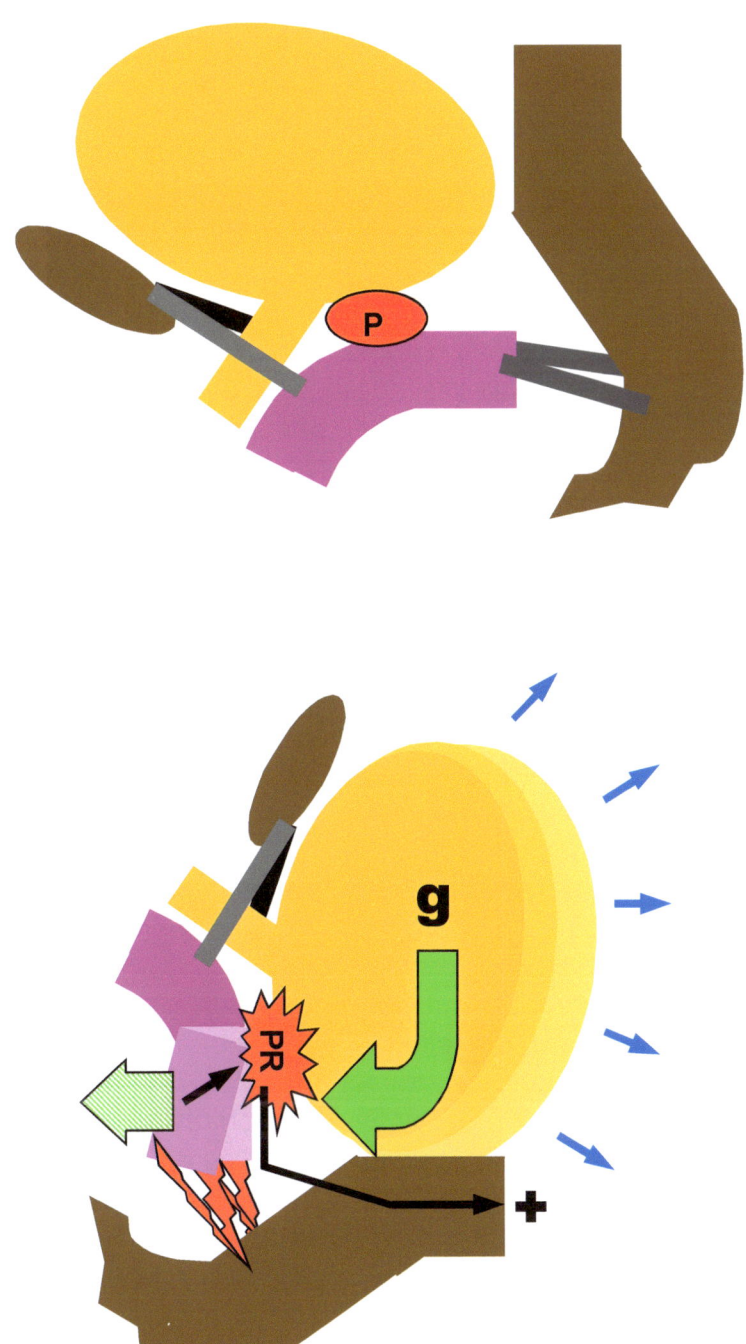

Fig. 15: The mechanism of induction of nocturia in women with bad uterosacral vault fixation or uterine descent due to looseness of USL

1.3.1.3 Detrusor instability (DI)

Laxity in all 3 zones may activate "Oa" the afferent limb of the micturition reflex (sensory urgency). CTX (Cortex), may respond by activating the neurological closure circuit "C". The suppression circuit "C" struggles for supremacy with the micturition circuit "O". Because of the time lag associated with feedback circuits, the detrusor instability graph characteristically demonstrates a phasic (bell shaped) pattern. Seen simplistically, as the micturition reflex "O" predominates, the detrusor contracts, and detrusor pressure rises. As "C" gradually wrests control of the neural pathways, the detrusor pressure falls back to the baseline. The spikes superimposed on the bell-shaped graph of detrusor instability represent the striated muscles of the external sphincter (Cm) contracting rapidly to try and close the urethra against the "open" phase. The manifestations of the micturition reflex were, in order of temporal occurrence: a sensation of urgency (sensory urgency), fall in urethral pressure (urethral instability), rise in detrusor pressure (detrusor instability), and urine loss (urge incontinence).

The decreasing yield, and time delay between each manifestation cause us to hypothesize that there may be at least 4 passes in the feedback loop, before urine is lost: sensory urgency (Oa), urethral relaxation (Ou), detrusor contraction (Od,) and finally, stretching open of the outflow tract by the pelvic floor muscles (Om). The underlying process may be similar for DI and normal micturition. A major anatomical defect preventing the action of Cm, may allow the backward opening forces (Om) to act as an accelerator (motor detrusor instability).

Note there is a time lag between urethral relaxation (Ou) and detrusor contraction(Od), and then follows a sudden acceleration in closure pressure fall at Om.

We know from video micturition studies that the urethra is always actively stretched open by pelvic floor contraction prior to urine loss, and we consider that in patients with DI, the same external muscle force acts as an accelerator for the micturition reflex (Om, figure 16). The detrusor contraction"Y" in the bottom graph "B", figure 16, has the classical bell-shaped curve of a feedback system; Om and urine loss were controlled at an early stage by "C", middle graph. As the detrusor continued to contract beyond the zone of urine loss (shaded area,bottom graph), we assume that control of urine loss was achieved by early activation of the peripheral control mechanism (Cm). This constricted the urethra, raised urethral resistance, and therefore, detrusor pressure. At the same time, the stretched vagina supported the urine column, decreasing the afferent stimulus from the stretch receptors, allowing the closure reflex "C" to predominate over "O", resulting in cessation of detrusor activity.

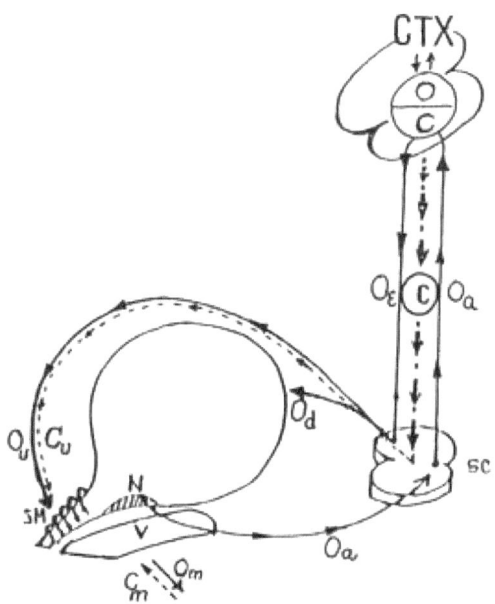

Figure 16 Schematic outline of central and peripheral control of the micturition reflex.
This is a sagittal simplified schematic representation of bladder, urethra, vagina, spinal cord (SC) and brain. "N"= nerve endings at bladder base, SM = intraurethral striated muscle sphincter. The broken lines represent the paths for closure"C". The unbroken lines "O" represent the paths of the micturition reflex - afferent outflow(Oa) from "N" to spinal cord and brain, and efferent flow(Oe) to detrusor(Od),urethra (Ou)and pelvic muscles (Om). CTX = cortex. The two directional arrows below vagina (V) represent the muscle forces acting during the micturition (Om) and closure (Cm) reflexes.

1.4 Stability of the Pelvic Floor System

Pelvic organ descent and prolapse develops due to deficiencies of the pelvic floor ligamentous and/or muscular structures.

The position of the pelvic organs are maintained in the pelvis by 3 main ways:

-muscular contraction
-fixation by ligaments
-the levator muscle forming a mechanical pressure-barrier.

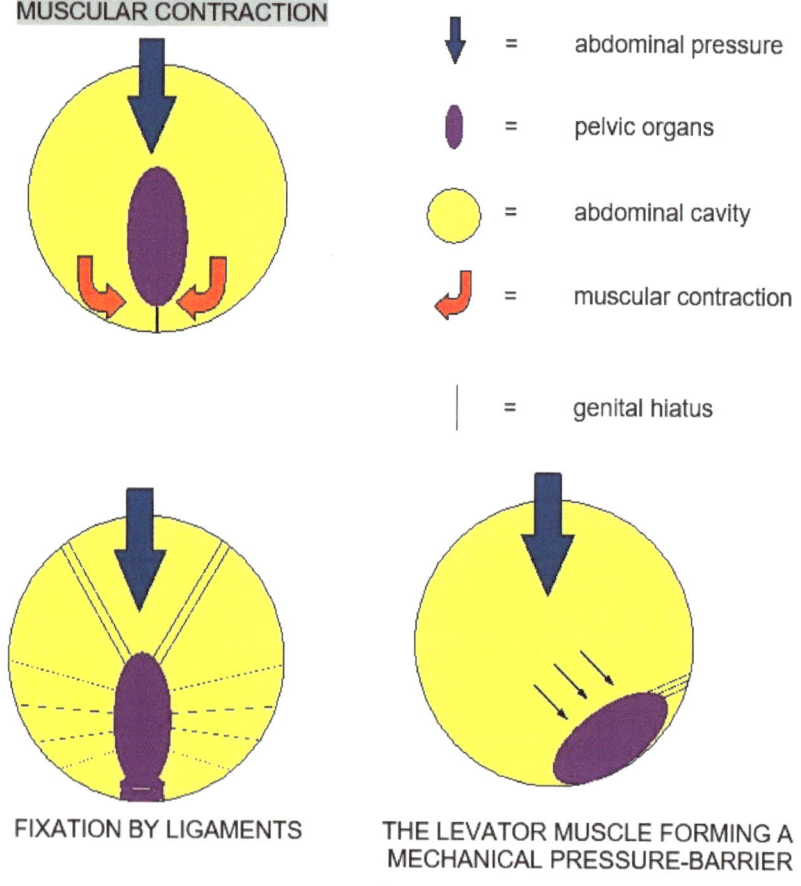

Fig. 17: Stability of the Pelvic Floor System (PFS)

According to DeLancey 3 criteria can be used to categorise defects into 3 levels as follows:

Muscular dysfunctions of the pelvic floor due to direct lesion, or secondary to neurogenic lesions are of great importance in the development of genital descent but do not readily respond (if at all) to surgical corrections such as the replacement of muscular structures by sutures or implants.

Neuro-muscular deficiency strains fascia and ligaments in a non-physiological way, causing secondary damage by excessive elongation and corresponding descent and malfunction.

Level	Fixation by	Anatomical structure	defect leads to...
Level 1	suspension	Parametrium/paracolpium	prolapse
Level 2	connection (tissue-mediated)	connection of vagina to arcus tendineous fasciae pelvis (Fascia pubocervicalis, Fascia rectovaginalis)	cystocele (lateral defect type)rectocele
Level 3	tensioning	direct fixation of vagina to surrounding structures by ligaments (Ligg. pubourethralia)	incontinence

Table 4: Stability of the PFS and ist disturbances

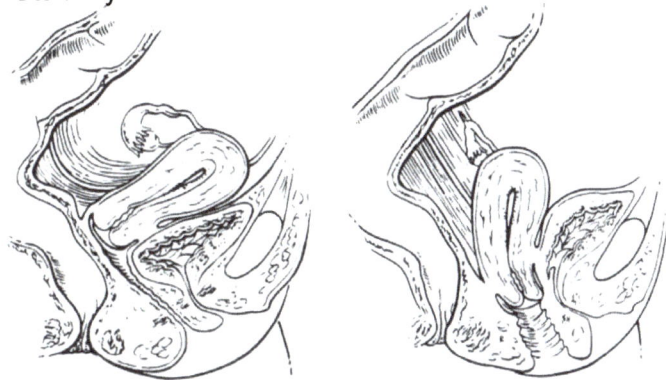

Fig. 18: Uterine prolapse

Such defects in ligaments and connective tissue integrity can however be effectively treated surgically. The posterior structures of relevance are:

-ureterosacral ligaments
-cardinal ligaments
-rectovaginal fascia (Denonvilliers) i.e. the rectovaginal layer of endopelvic fascia and, connected to the rectovaginal fascia, is the tendinous centre of the perineum (the fusion of both halves of the transverse perineal muscle and the bulbocavernous muscle).

The perineal body is reinforced by the continuation of the rectovaginal fascia which separates the anorectum from the vaginal vestibule. It is a weakening of this bulkhead that significantly reduces the stability of bladder, rectum, uterus and perineum.

There are numerous disorders, and combinations of disorders, of the endopelvic fascia and/or ligaments connecting or interconnecting the organs to the pelvic wall.
The concept of their treatment is:

- strengthening of the muscle forces
- support of the vaginal walls compensating for connective tissue laxity
- support of thje mid-urtethra to ensure continence

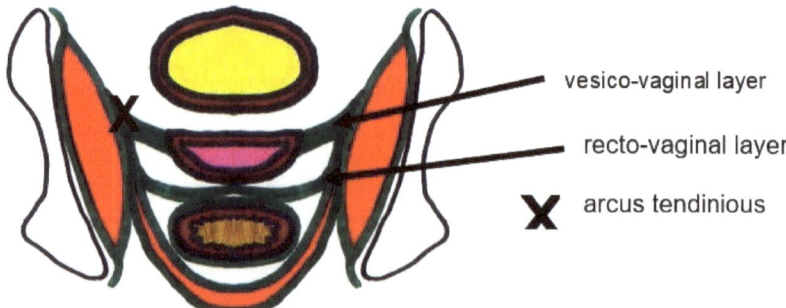

Fig. 19: Pelvic floor fascia

1.5 Anterior Vaginal wall defects

Are one of the most frequent and obvious defects we encounter.
When managing a cystocoele and choosing the optimum surgical intervention we have to distinguish between a midline defect (a tear in the pubocervical layer of the endopelvic fascia) and a unilateral or bilateral lateral defect (caused by the detachment of the vagina from the arcus tendinious)

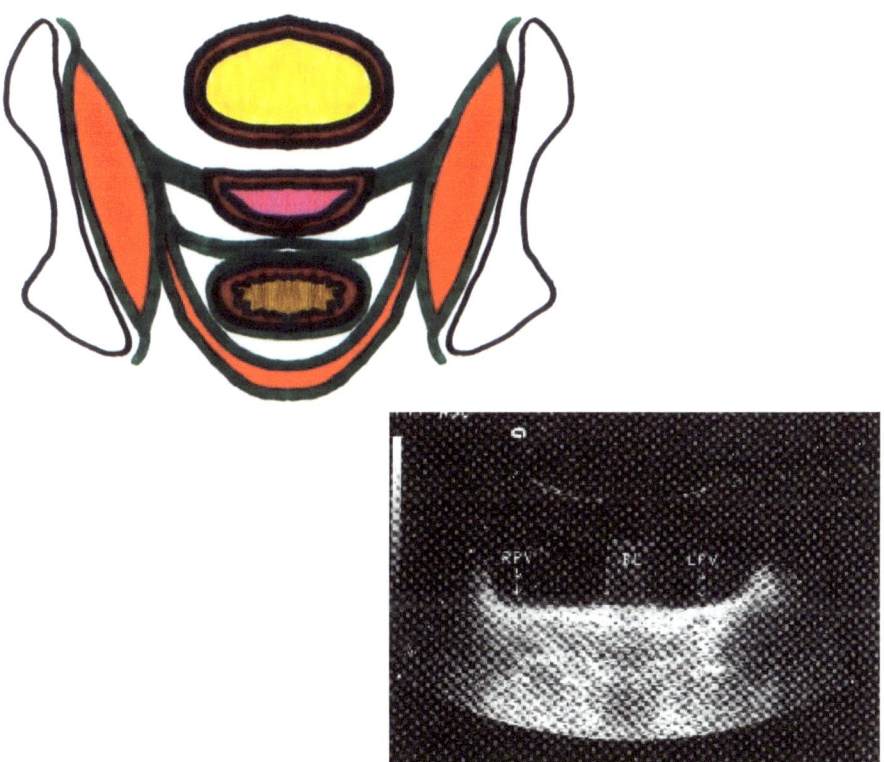

Figure 20: Normal anatomy and abdominal sono-anatomy of lateral vaginal

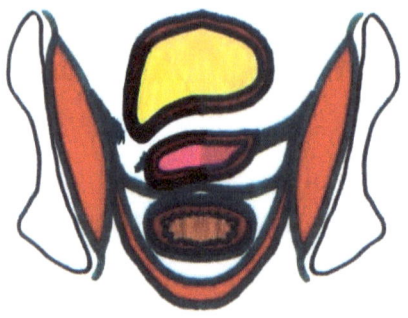 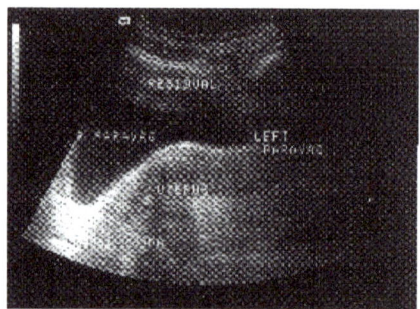

Figure 21: Anatomy and abdominal sonoanatomy in unilateral detachment of the vagina

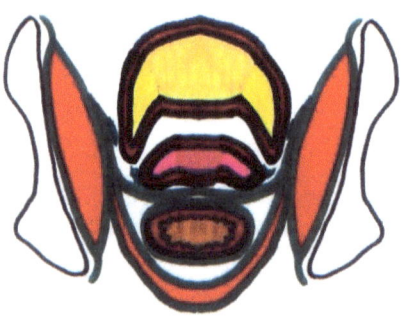 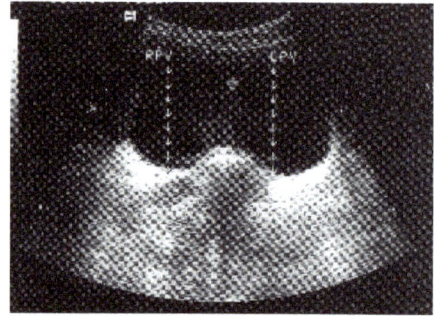

Figure 22: Anatomy and abdominal sonoanatomy in bilateral vaginal detachment

1.5.1 The midline defect (Fig. 23)

is diagnosed upon inspection of the anterior vaginal wall where the rugae vaginales have disappeared in the area of the distension but are intact in the lateral aspects (sulci laterales).

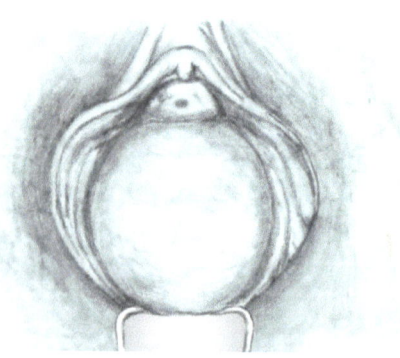

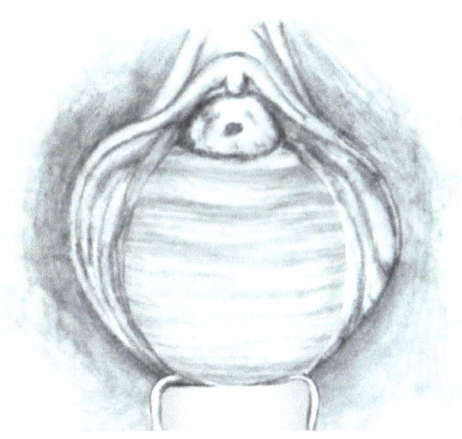

Fig. 24: The lateral defect shows either a descent, or virtual disappearance of, the lateral vaginal sulcus with intact rugae.

1.5.2 Lateral Defect

Incorrectly treating the lateral defect as if it were a midline defect would means further separating the fascial edges of the tear and hereby enlarging the hernia. Plication of the intact fascia in the midline for treatment of a uni– or bilateral defect therefore worsens the lateral detachment, increasing the defect, however this remains the standard procedure in many centres.

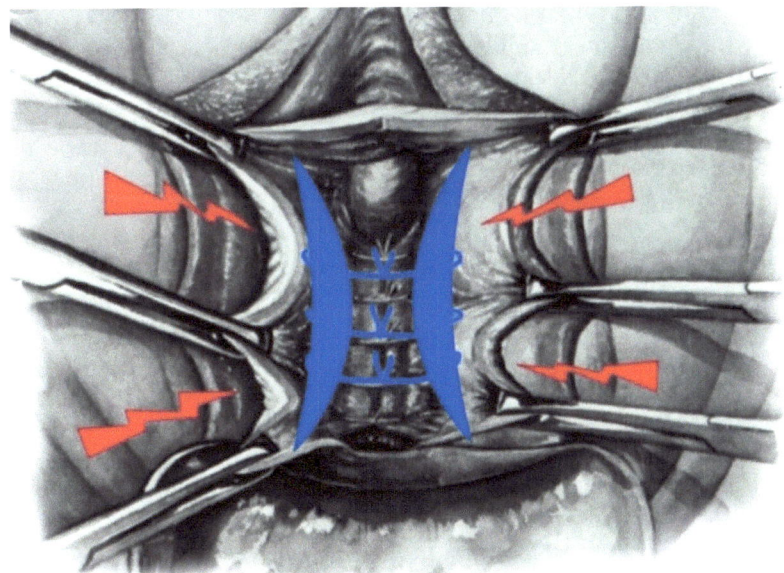

Fig. 25: Effect of midline conventional repair on lateral fixation of the endopelvic fascia

Fig. 26: Different types of prolapse

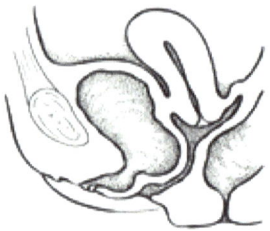

Lateral defect-type of cystocele
Distension or tear of the connection between endopelvic fascia and ATFP (arcus tendineous fasciae pelvis) at the pelvic wall level

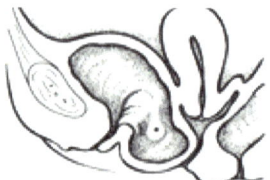

Midline-typ of cystocele
Distension or tear in the connective tissue layer underneath the bladder base - vesico-vaginal layer of the endopelvic fascia

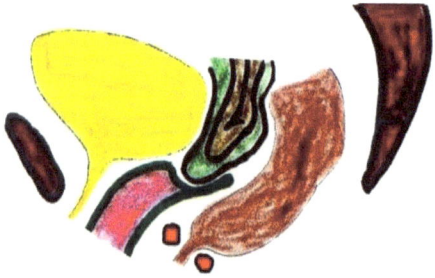

Anterior enterocele
After removal of the uterus the small intestine may form an enterocele above the apical scar tissue or attachement of the vault applying pressure to the bladder base (which may result in urgency)

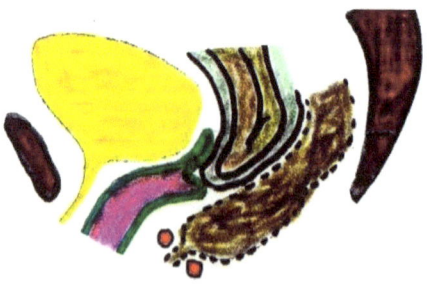

Posterior enterocele
More common, the small intestine squeezes in the space between uterus/vault and anterior rectum wall causing defecation difficulties

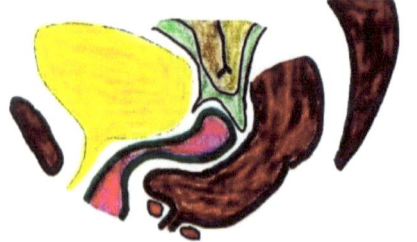

Rectocele
Distension of the anterior rectum wall caused by connective tiussue defects at various levels (midline, lateral

1.6 Posterior Vaginal Wall Defects

1.6.1 Rectocele
In a rectocele the vaginal wall herniation contains the extended ampoule of the rectum. The defect of the rectovaginal layer of the endopelvic fascia can be located in the midline, laterally or transversally near the vaginal entry.
The symptoms of a distension of vagina and rectum often lead to a dehydrated stool and constipation.
The connective tissue of this fascial layer is very thin so we have to consider alternatives to restore stability. Interposition of the levator muscle is the most common technique although this dislocation of the muscle often causes a tight vaginal vestibule with dyspareunia, pain and anorectal dysfunction.
Figure 27 showing recto- (27a) and enterocele (27b/c) being difficult to treat tension-free without using tissue replacement.

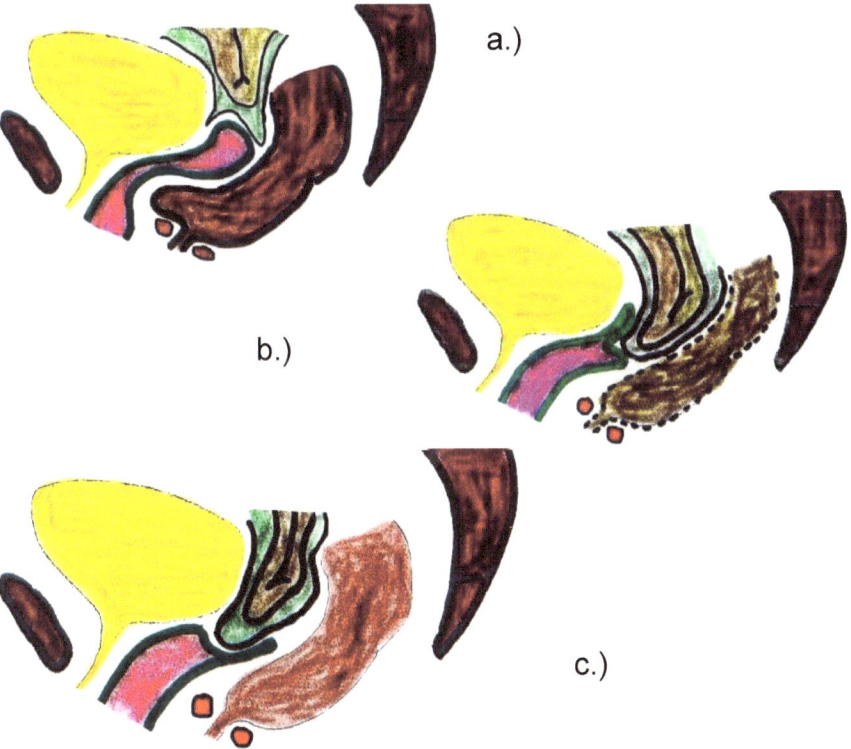

Fig. 27: Forms of posterior defect

1.6.2 Enterocele

The enterocele contains a protrusion of the peritoneum containing the small intestine.

Excessive formation of scar tissue in the lower parts of the vagina (caused by childbirth or previous surgery) may lead to an enterocele in the absence of a rectocele but in most patients recto– and enterocele, appear in tandem.

A protrusion of the small intestine may also appear in the upper part of the anterior vaginal wall, camouflaged as a cystocele in cases with a fairly good suspended vaginal apex. Inspection sometimes gives a hint when the bowels movement can be seen through the vaginal wall. although sometimes perineal ultrasound or lateral cysturethrography are needed to distinguish the true cystocele from the anterior upper enterocele.

The protruding enterocele mainly causes rubbing, chafing, excoriation and the feeling of a foreign body in the vagina or between the legs.

There is no tissue in this region which to plicate or to fix to any of the pelvic wall structures.

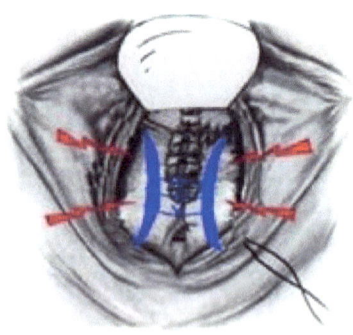

Fig. 28: Tear location of posterior endopelvic fascia and effect of plication

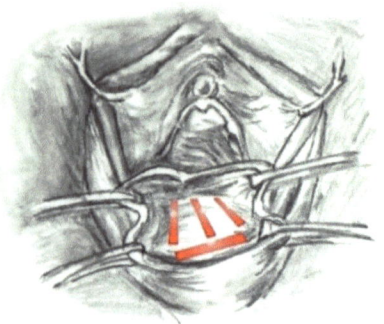

Chapter 2 Basics of Conservative Treatment

2.1 Hormones – Oestrogens (Fig. 29)

When reaching menopause the ovaries significantly reduce their hormone production. Hot flush and depressive mood are commonly known to be its symptoms as well as osteoporosis and arteriosclerosis. Important changes also occur (sometimes earlier than flush and moods) at the level of vaginal skin, urethral and bladder mucosa. They are getting thinner, loose their lubrication and becoming more sensitive and damageable leading to dyspareunia and irritation of the above mentioned tissues resulting in itching, bleeding, reduction of vaginal pH value, infections of vagina and bladder, urgency and reduction of stress continence.

Therefore local oestrogens are of the utmost importance in women when approaching menopause. We recommend 0.5 mg Estriol twice a week locally (two halves of a 1 mg tablet),

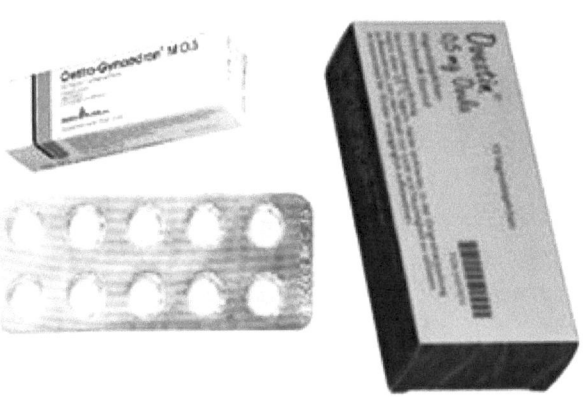

suppositories are also available but cause itching, burning and vaginal discharge in too many cases so that patient's compliance is not as good as with tablets.

Estriol leads to an increased turn-over-rate of superficial vaginal epithelial cells used by lactobacillus to produce lactic acid. The vaginal pH value drops and with that the infection rate of vagina and bladder. Thicker epithelial tissue layers, better lubrication, increased perfusion, reduced rigidity are also effects of local Estriol application.

There are no contraindications in patients with diabetes, varicosis, hyprtension, hyperlipaemia and specialists even recommend low-dosage local application (up to 0.03 mg per day) in patients with breastcancer as the absorption rate of locally applied Estriol is extremely low. That also implicates that there is no significant effect on other menopausal symptoms.

2.2 Treament with PVA-Tampons (Contam®)

Contam tampons or plugs are a subtype of the large family of genital pessaries.
Tampons made of PVA (Poylvinylalcohol) can be used for different purposes:
- Stress urinary incontinence
- Urge incontinence due to instability at bladder-base or bladder-neck level
- Prolapse
- For preop. Treatment
- As an alternative to surgical treatment
- Treatment of postop. vaginal scars
- Protection of surgical result after pelvic floor surgery

(especially with continuous strain on pelvic flor i. e. due to work

Insertion of these soft foam-based tampons needs a little less skill than needed for the insertion of silicone-based (cubic) pessaries. They can be re-used when properly cleaned and give a good comfort when correctly brought into position. The risk of dislocation depends on the amount of prolapse and the quality of the pelvic floor muscles.

In most patients we recommend the insertion in the morning after the morning toilet using a little Estriol cream. They can be cleaned with warm water during the day should the need arise and then re-inserted or their position can be rectified in cases of dislocation. Before bedtime they are removed, cleaned with warm water and afterwards rinsed with diluted vinegar.

Using the tampons 6-8 times (with a day between applications to ensure complete drying) and inserting them using a little Estriol cream irritations and inflammations of the vagina are very rare.

There are also anal plugs available to be used in patients with anal incontinence. They come in different shapes and sizes.

The advantages of PVA-Tampons are:
- Soft, tender, elastic
- Not visible
- Individually fittable
- Reduce odours
- Multiple usage possible (if wished).

The drilling of the tampon in it centre allows the patient to use an applicator for its insertion, which makes the correct positioning much easier especially in slightly obese women. The possibility to command individually confected tampons (length range from 3 - 5.5 cm) leads to an even better satisfaction of different patient's needs.

Available Tampons

1.) Classic form
Treatment of Stress Urinary Incontinence (SUI) (loss of urine when coughing, laughing, lifting things,...), to activate and strengthen pelvic floor muscles, to prevent or delay surgery, to stabilize postop. results, to prevent progress while excersising

2.) Cube-shaped form
Treatment of prolapse (uterus, vagina [bladder, rectum]], SUI, Urgency whgen causes by hypermobility of anterior vaginal wall. Treatment of scartissue.

All tampons are made for self treatment.

3.) Contam Duo
I scarecely use them. They are supposed to better support the urethra than the standard shape.

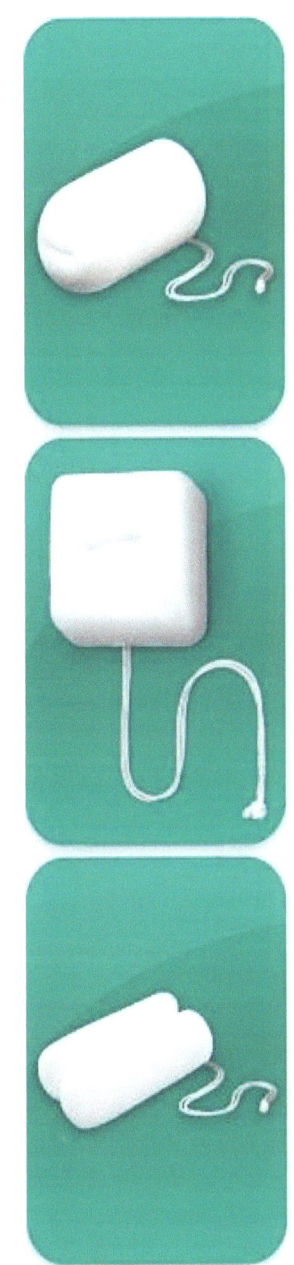

Fig. 30: Available Tampons (Contam®)

4.) **Contam Special**
The indications are the same as for the standard tampons. The groove shape allows more cream to be applied to the vaginal skin.

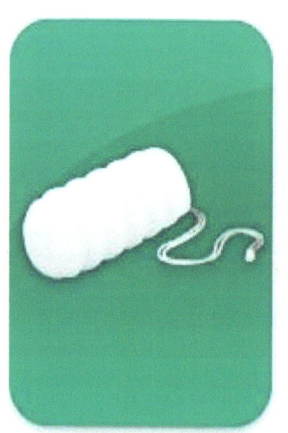

5.) **Contam Med**
The indications are the same as for the standard tampons. The groove shape allows more cream to be applied to the vaginal skin. The longitudinal groove spares the urethra from the tampons pressure if with standard plugs micturition is disturbed by the tampons pressure tu the urethra.

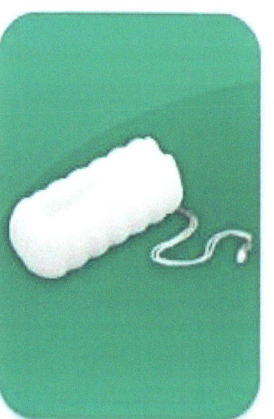

6.) **PVA-Anal plugs**
For anal incontinence there is a large variety of different plugs suiting the patient's need.

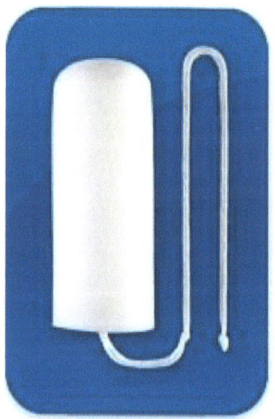

Fig. 31: Available Tampons (Contam®)

The drilling of the tampon in it centre allows the patient to use an applicator for its insertion, which makes the correct positioning much easier especially in slightly obese women. The possibility to command individually confected tampons (length range from 3 - 5.5 cm) leads to an even better satisfaction of different patient's needs.

Available Tampons

1.) Classic form
Treatment of Stress Urinary Incontinence (SUI) (loss of urine when coughing, laughing, lifting things,...), to activate and strengthen pelvic floor muscles, to prevent or delay surgery, to stabilize postop. results, to prevent progress while excersising

2.) Cube-shaped form
Treatment of prolapse (uterus, vagina [bladder, rectum]], SUI, Urgency whgen causes by hypermobility of anterior vaginal wall. Treatment of scartissue.

All tampons are made for self treatment.

3.) Contam Duo
I scarecely use them. They are supposed to better support the urethra than the standard shape.

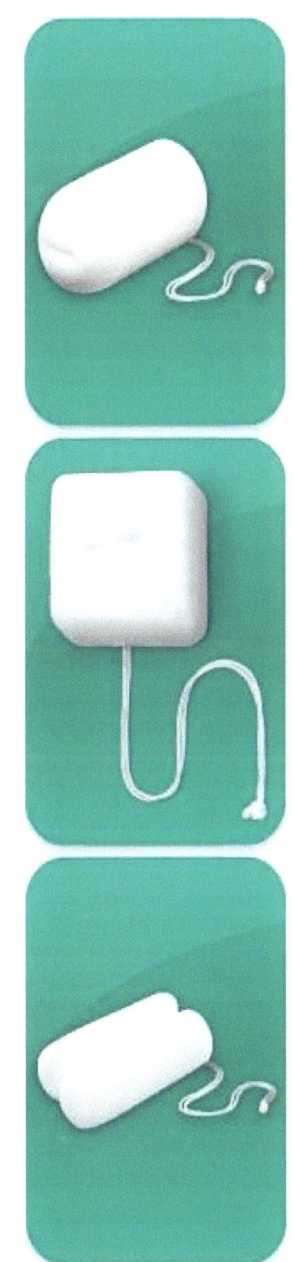

Fig. 30: Available Tampons (Contam®)

4.) Contam Special
The indications are the same as for the standard tampons. The groove shape allows more cream to be applied to the vaginal skin.

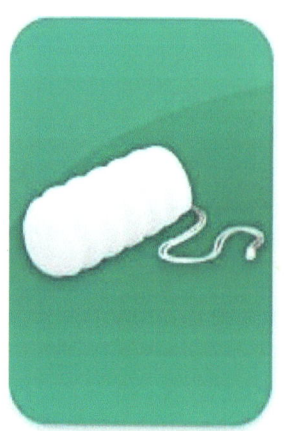

5.) Contam Med
The indications are the same as for the standard tampons. The groove shape allows more cream to be applied to the vaginal skin. The longitudinal groove spares the urethra from the tampons pressure if with standard plugs micturition is disturbed by the tampons pressure tu the urethra.

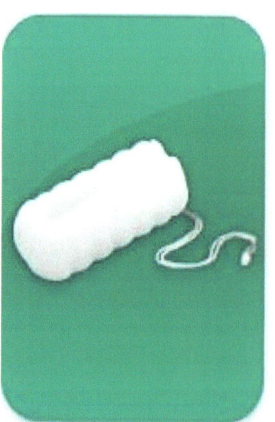

6.) PVA-Anal plugs
For anal incontinence there is a large variety of different plugs suiting the patient's need.

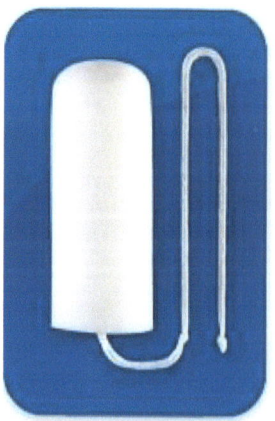

Fig. 31: Available Tampons (Contam®)

Left:
6a.) Cylindrical form
In cases with residual function of the external sphincter ani muscle (SAE) in analogy to the use of gynaecological tampons

6b.) Concave form
Suits the needs of the anal closing system in cases of reduced tonus and contraction of the SAE.

6c.) spherical form
Works like a ball valve in cases with no residual function of the SAE to close off the ampulla recti.

6d.) spiral form
The grooves work like channels to release gases in cases with mild diarrhoea and improves stability when positioned.

Right:
6 e.) cone form
The ball valve part closes off the rectum, the middle part supports a residual SAE function

6f.) Convex form
Works like 6e without the ball valve part of 6e

6g.) Anal safety device
Secures the tampon and prevents its dislocation/expulsion

6h.) Applicators
To facilitate the tampon's insertion

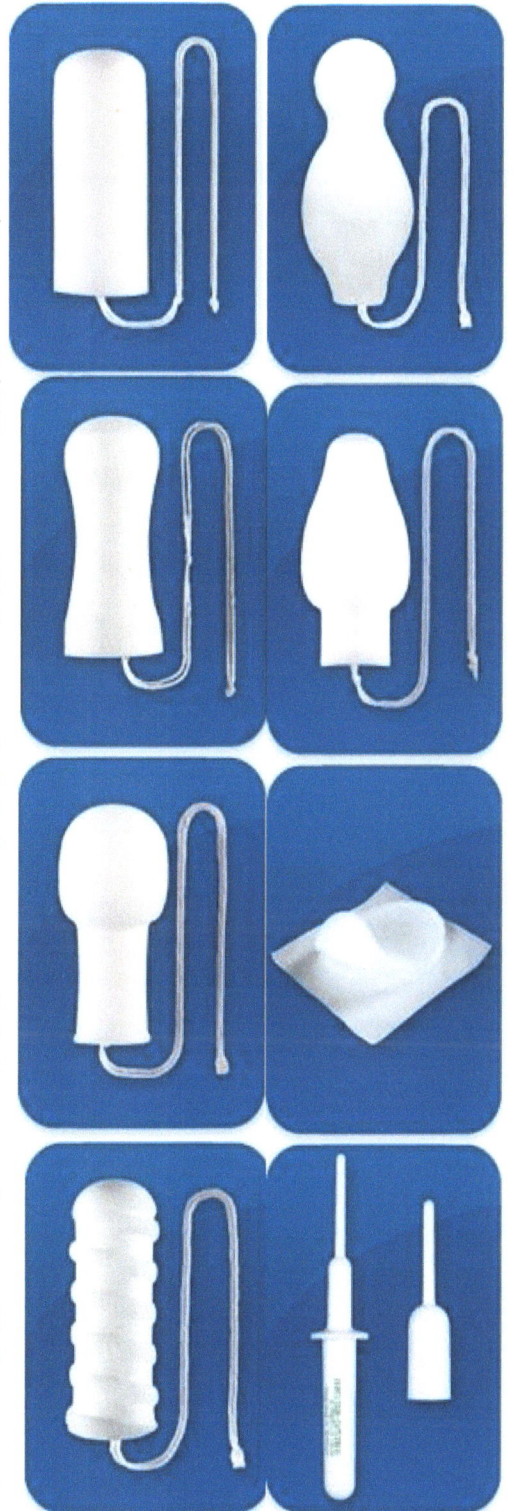

Fig. 32: Available Tampons/Aids (Contam®)

2.3 Pessary Treatment

Many women think that pessary treatment is something old-fashioned or even obsolete. Not true! In former times pessaries remained in the vagina for a few weeks before being removed, cleaned and re-inserted. This is still an option with very old ladies or those who do not wish a self-treatment. But even then infections, ulcers or bleeding are very rare. Sometimes women forget about their pessaries. Those cases can cause severe infections or ulcers. This is why we recommend and support self-treatment.

Pessaries are devices to restore vaginal anatomy and/or function and are made of silicone. They come in different shapes and sizes to fit the patient's needs. In most cases the patient inserts it in the morning (after defecation) and removes the pessary before going to bed, then rinsing it with warm water to let it dry over night. Some patients remove it every tow, three or even seven days, some only wear it during the night. This demonstrates a highly flexible treatment to the needs of the patient. Most pessaries have to be removed before intercourse.

The role of the gynaecologist is to chose the right pessary-type and the best-fitting size. The majority of patients use an estriol cream for insertion. Detergents for cleaning are not allowed, remainders may disturb the vaginal flora.

The duration of pessary treatment depends on the patient's satisfaction with the treatment, the efficacy and other options in treatment. In some cases they are predecessors to surgery, in others surgery becomes unnecessary with an effective pessary treatment.

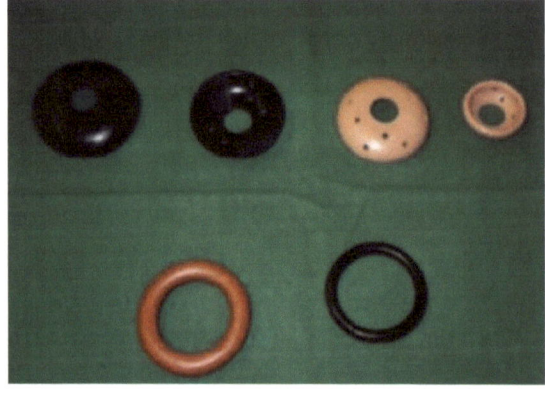

Fig. 33: Forms of circular pessaries

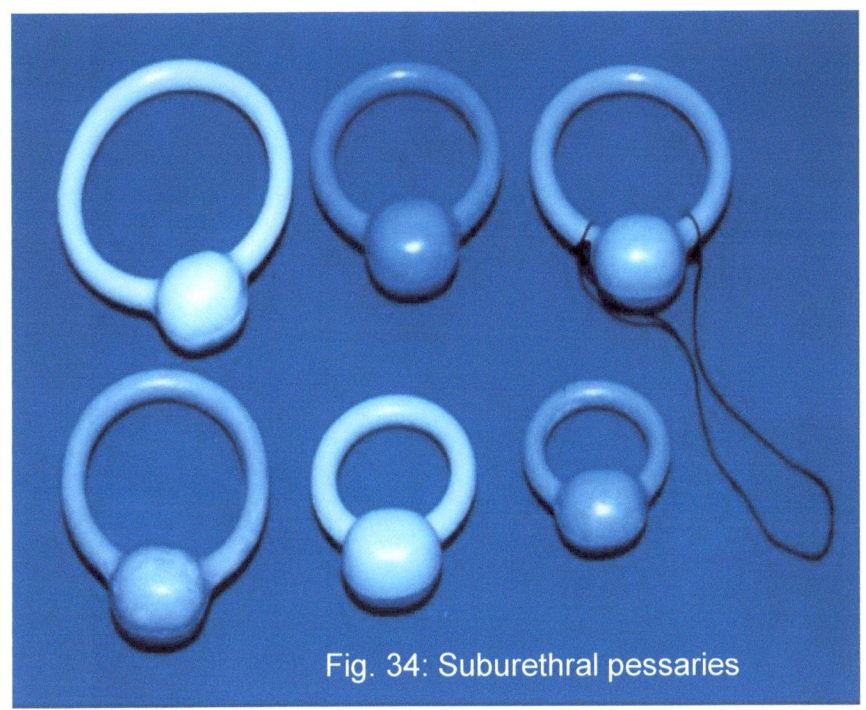

Fig. 34: Suburethral pessaries

2.3.1 The use of ring-shaped pessaries

The ring-form with its suburethral pelotte is mainly used in stress urinary incontinence. Resting on the levator ani muscle the pelotte supports and slightly compresses the urethra with the rise of the abdominal pressure ensuring a better closure pressure and hence continence. The supporting muscle is at the same time stimulated to contract which is part of an internal pelvic floor muscle re-education.

The pessaries can be worn either all day long or for periods of elevated strain on the pelvic floor (work, sport, …). In some cases it is recommendable to wear it during the night (nocturia) or even a few days in a row. It does not disturb or hinder micturition and has not to be removed. Sometimes (with rectoceles) defecation may cause dislocation and necessitate a re-insertion or adjustment afterwards.

After removal they only have to be rinsed with fairly hot water and then left to dry on their own. No detergents should be used to clean a pessary because its remainders will disturb the vaginal flora.

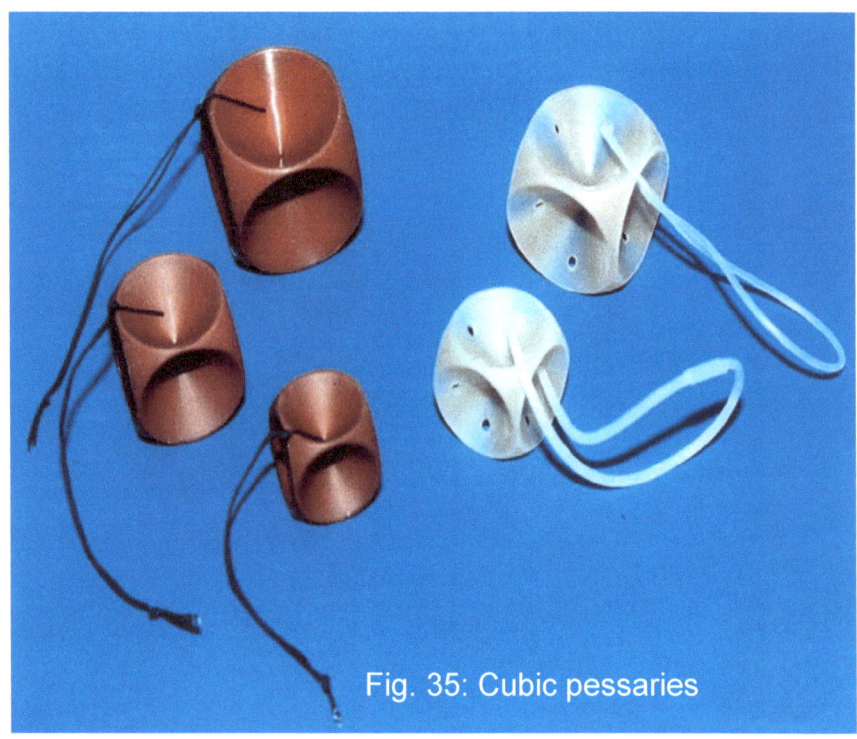

Fig. 35: Cubic pessaries

2.3.2 The use of cubic pessaries

Cubes are mainly used for prolapse, in some cases when rings are difficult or impossible to place or to be kept in a good position (i. e. after hysterectomy) also for urinary incontinence but they are also quite valuable to detect a hidden urinary incontinence due to urethral kinking as a result of a cystocele that causes the urethra to be closed by the kink at the level of the urethra's fixation (by pubourethral ligament i.e.).

The surface of the cube is able to create a vacuum which assures a secure position even in cases with larger cysto- or rectoceles (as long as there is sufficient pelvic flor muscle to support the cube's edges).

In some cases cubes can be used to soften scar tissue after surgery and lengthen or widen the vagina when using different sizes (from very small (size 0) to larger sizes (up to size 2, 3 or 4).

During pregnancy the perforated cubes can ease the stress on the pelvic floor during week 16 and 28.

Fig. 36: Pessary Treatment

A: Urethra Pessaries by Arabin
B: Cube Pessaries by Arabin
C: Urethral pessary in urinary stress incontinence (SUI)
D: Cubic pessary in prolapse (left) and SUI (right)
E: how to insert a pessary (above right "Ring", below "Cube")

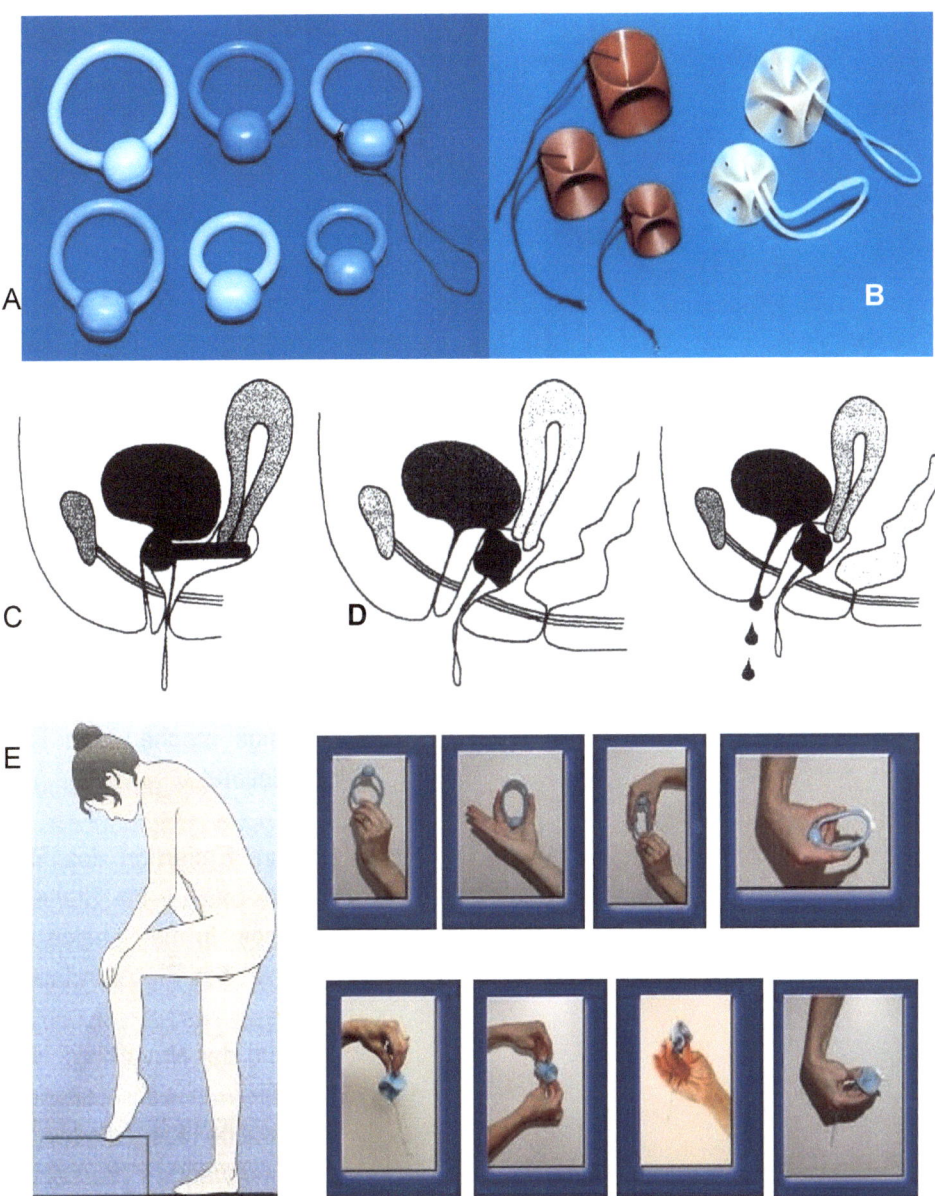

3.4 Pelvic Floor Physiotherapy

Pelvic floor physiotherapy is one of the basic pillars of pelvic floor disorder treatment. Main goals are to teach the perception of pelvic floor muscle contraction, to maintain the masses of working pelvic floor muscles and to train women to protect the system when working or exercising and in the perception of the muscles' activities. The physiotherapist hast to teach the patient in the perception and use of the pelvic floor muscle, coaching the re-education and supervise the patient's efforts.

It is possible to do pelvic floor exercises in groups, we recommend to start with an individual setting to work more individually and intensely to the individual's needs. Cooperation between urogynaecologist and physiotherapist is of the utmost importance for the patient's success.

It is desirable to have a physiotherapist who is trained in vaginal examination to evaluate the progress of pelvic floor muscle training in the patient. The evaluation can be documented using the following schemes:

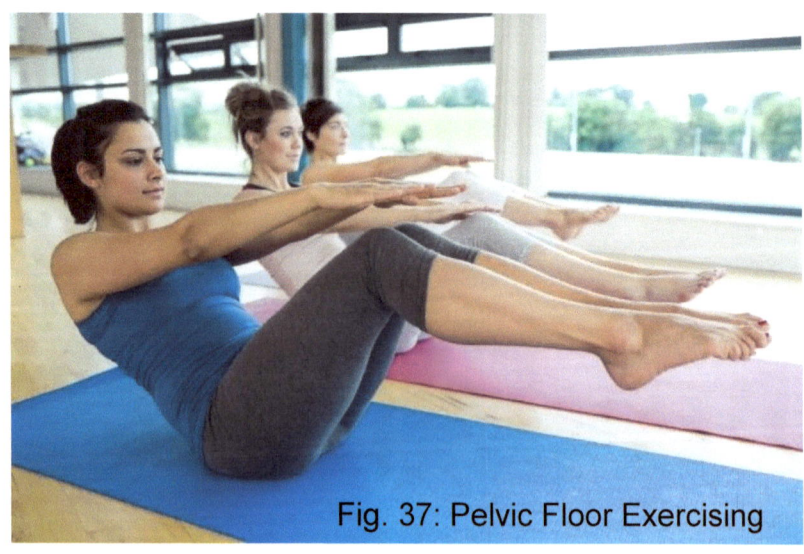

Fig. 37: Pelvic Floor Exercising

P	Power	Power of the contraction, cf. Oxford Grading
E	Endurance	keep tension approximately for 10 sec., then relax (slow-twitch fibers)
R	Repetitions	approximately 5 repetitions, then relax
F	Fast Contractions	10 fast contractions (fast-twitch fibers)
E	Elevation	testing the „lift" of the levator ani muscle
C	Cough Response	contractions with cough ? Loss of urine?
T	Transcribe it all	write results down to compare later

Tab.5: Above: PERFECT-Scheme according to Laycock 1994
Tab. 6: Below: Oxford-Grading

Grade	Muscle function
0	no contraction
1	flicker of non-sustained contraction
2	presence of low intensitiy, but sustained contraction
3	moderate contraction, small cranial elevation of the vagina and very soft compression of the examiner's fingers
4	satisfactory contracion, compression of fingers and elevation of vagina towards the pubic symphysis
5	strong contraction, firm compression of the examiner's fingers with positive movement towards symphysis

It is advisable to examine and score the pelvic floor before, during and after the first series of pelvic floor exercises, regardless of what form of therapy is used to re-educate it.

Fig. 38: Physiotherapist explaining the Pelvic floor using pictures and a mirror

a) Examination in upright position I

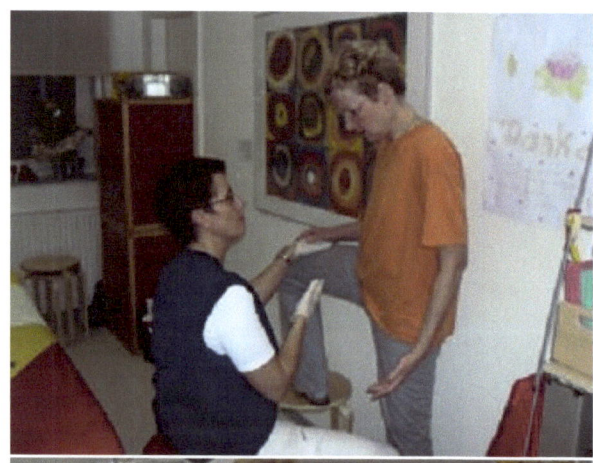

b) Examination in upright position II

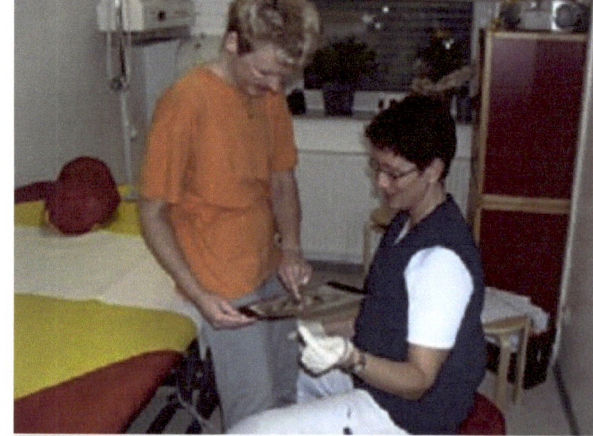

c) Mirror-controlled feedback sitting down

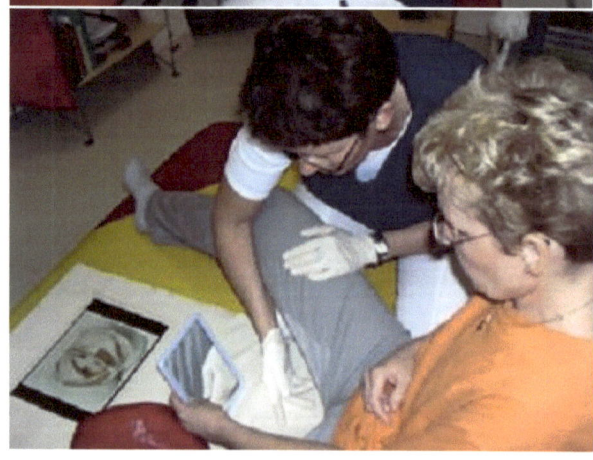

Fig. 39 (left): Loveballs and Laycock-Device

Fig. 39 (right): Rose quarz-eggs

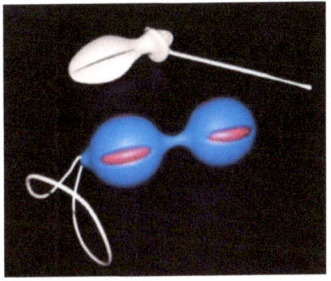
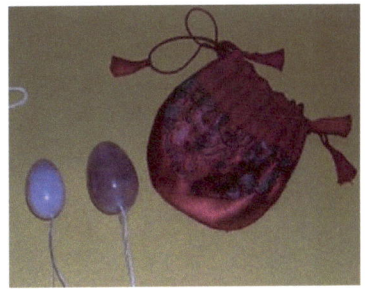

Physiotherapy starts with a talk about micturition habits, position and frequency of micturition and defecation. The earlier the better. We think that pelvic floor education should start in school.

Not only the weak pelvic floor needs attention but also the tense one, often due to a fear to lose urine. This is also very important for the patient's sex life. A good pelvic floor coordination is the main goal of physiotherapy.

Building-up the muscle cannot be achieved by pelvic floor exercises (also called Kegel exercises), this can sufficiently only achieved by electric myostimulation (see next chapter). The middle frequency band, modulated, is more efficient than low-band stimulation and apparently external stimulation with modulated middle frequency currents reaches a larger volume of muscle in the depth of the pelvis.

The physiotherapist should try to train slow- and fast twitch fibers as well as perception, contraction and relaxation of the pelvic floor. Micturition and defecation training should be included in the program, especially when there is an erratic behaviour noticed by the physiotherapist. Prolapse situations are especially challenging and should be treated in cooperation with the urogynecologist. The use of devices (fig. above) may be advisable to enhance perception and effectiveness of contraction or relaxation exercises. Pessaries can also be necessary to better train the muscles. Last but not least the patient should have at least a little fun doing the exercises, the compliance improves when exercising is not perceived as a burden but as something worthwhile.

Part II
Electrotherapy

3.1 Conventional Electrophysiotherapy

Electrotherapy of the pelvic floor is a well established treatment and can be administered in SUI and urgency (UI) leading to improvement in approximately 1/3 of the urge patients and in up to 50% in patients with SUI.

The focus of electro-"stimulation" as it often called seems to be the pudendal nerve (for SUI) and the N. pelvicus (for UI), stimulating the former and inhibiting the latter. In low frequency treatment the results improve with reduced distance to the pudendal nerve hence using intravaginal or intraanal electrodes. The pelvic nerve can also be stimulated by pre-sacral or pre-pubic skin electrodes. In most of the cases it is advisable to accompany this form of treatment with conventional physiotherapy as described in the last chapter. The needed devices can be prescribed and used at home at least every second day. The following counterindications should be respected:

- Pregnancy
- Bleeding disorders
- Inflammations of the vulva or vagina
- Urinary tract infections
- Growing uterus due to fibroids
- Urinary retention
- Severe cardiac arrhythmia
- Pacemaker.

Different current frequencies can be used in electrotherapy

frequency	used with….
Low frequency current	
Transcutaneous electric nerve stimulation (TENS) 10-100 Hz 10-20 Hz – short- time stimulation 50 Hz long-time stimulation	Sensoric urgency, urethral syndrome, irritable bladder disorder Motor-urge (idiopathic) SUI
10-20/50 Hz stimulation	SUI, UI
Middle frequency current (interference current)	SUI, UI (in older patients)
High frequency current (short-, microwave)	Improvement of perfusion, relaxation in the detrusor-sphincter-unity

Table 7: Use of different current frequencies

3.2 Biofeedback Therapy

The registration of muscular activity applying vaginal or anal probes can be used to demonstrate the effects of the patient's efforts to contract or relax the pelvic floor by lights and/or sound. The registered currents (µV) depend on the devices and are not comparable. This form of therapy can be used in SUI, UI and Faecal (Anal) Incontinence.

Power of activity, endurance and elapsed time from contracting to achieving a contraction can be registered and used in therapy. The training period should extend over 20-30 minutes per day. To avoid mass contractions of surrounding muscles the initiation should be accompanied by a physiotherapist. After 12-16 weeks the patient should be seen by the prescribing physician.

Contraindications are
- Lack of compliance
- Menstruation
- Urinary tract infection
- Uncertainty of the insufficiency's cause
- Physical or mental disabilities of the patient interfering with the handling of the device.

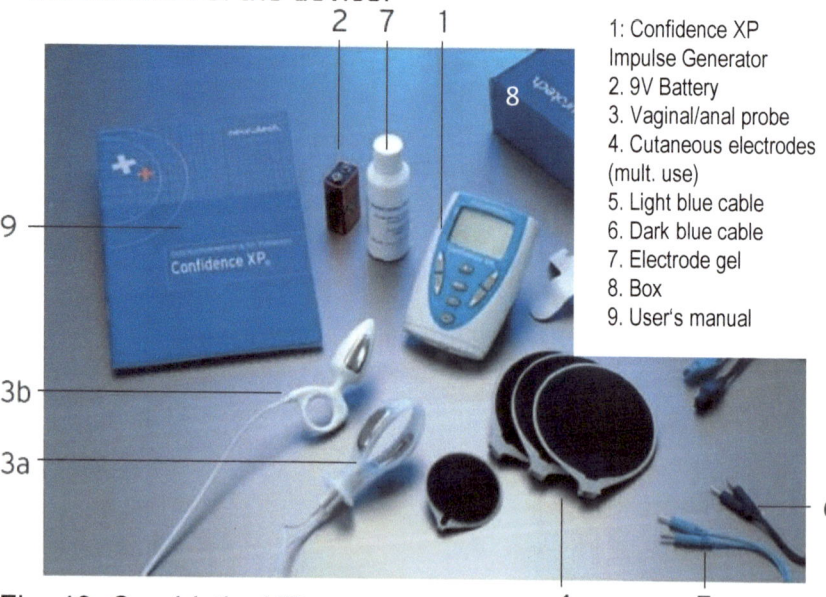

1: Confidence XP Impulse Generator
2. 9V Battery
3. Vaginal/anal probe
4. Cutaneous electrodes (mult. use)
5. Light blue cable
6. Dark blue cable
7. Electrode gel
8. Box
9. User's manual

Fig. 40: Combistim XP

3.3 External Electric Muscle Activation (EEMA)

Exercising with the use of electric current is very popular and well commercialised claiming that the current used, low frequency in most cases, is more effective and time preserving than conventional fitness training.

It is hence only obvious that electric muscular stimulation (EMS) should be used to train the pelvic floor as well. But low frequency current externally applied is not as effective as middle frequency current. There are some major differences in the biological effect of those two types of current:
- The volume reached (in the depth of the pelvis) is larger with MFC (middle frequency current)
- MFC does not induce pain or muscle soreness while or after exercising
- MFC activates the cell's metabolism and the increase in volume is more significant than with LFC (low frequency current).

We therefore chose a distinction between
- EMS – a term that can be generally applied describing this form of treatment, but often referring to LFC
- (E)EMA – a term we only use when modulated MFC is applied to the body. The first "E" stands for "External" because the current is externally administered

If combined with special exercises the efficacy of the treatment improves and the parts of the pelvic floor muscle that comes into focus can be variated. This is important in cases where parts of the muscle are damaged.

Fig. 41: StimaWell EMS

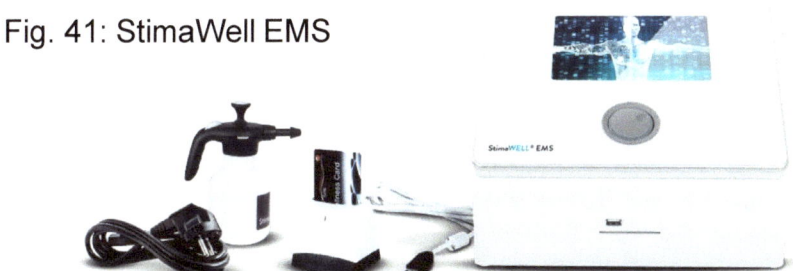

LFC stimulates the muscle provoking a contractive response by the muscle cell(s). One impulse leads to one action potential of the muscle cell up to a frequency where the next impulse falls into the absolute refractory period of the muscle cell.

MFC does not directly stimulate the cell because of the high frequency of impulses. It directly activates the muscle cell leaving it the choice to react with a contraction if ready without stimulating the connected nerve and thereby not causing unpleasing/painful sensations.

By modulating the impulses created by a far more complex impulse generator than needed for LFC-stimulation (and therefore more expensive) effect, depth and volume stimulated can be varied. The effect of stimulation resembles very much the biological activation of the muscle when the signal is appropriately pure (which depends on the quality of the generator).

EMA works with a 2 kHz carrier wave with pure rectangular impulses even in the depth of the tissue onto which low frequency impulses can be added (modulated) to achieve the desired effects caused by LFC (relaxation pain reduction, contraction as a growth stimulus for the muscle.

The often used term "myomodulation" is used to show that the electric impulse does not reach the muscle cell via its nerve fibre but is directly stimulate the the muscle cells sarcolemma (syn. myolemma, the cell membrane of the striated muscle fibre cell). The sarcolemma does not dispose of a myolin sheath so that there is no saltatoric progression of the impulse, which slows down the impulse's transmission compared to the n significantly compared to the motoneuron. The impulse generator has to administer to those needs. It is a quasi-physiological effect of the modulated MFC that helps to train more units than with LFC stimulating the motoneuron itself but not the muscle fibres directly.

A side effect is the increase of bowel peristalsis, something very useful in most women's slow transit of defecation disorders.

3.3.1 Modulated Middle Frequency Electrotherapy (MFT, EEMA)

We see the modulated MFC treatment as a very important piece of the pelvic floor's therapy puzzle and wish to dedicate the following chapter to this not yet very widely spread form of electrophysiotherapy.

EEMA combines the benefits of LFC and MFC without combining or adding their disadvantages.

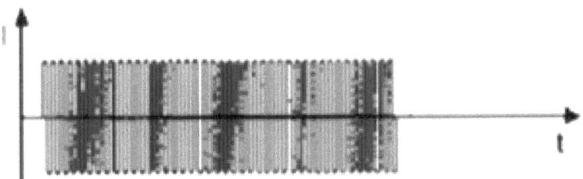

Fig. 42: Sinus-shaped MFC (f= 1000 waves per second (Hz), t(i)= 0.5 sec

In EEMA we use a rectangular-shaped MFC of 2-6 kHz as a carrier wave to pass through the large volume of muscular tissue due to the Gildemeister effect and the Wedensky inhibition (s. below). EEMA's main effects are:
- continuous activation
- Pain reduction due to permanent depolarization inhibiting the nerve fibres to fire (chronic pain)
- Direct stimulation of the muscle to improve activity and mass

Onto the carrier wave we can modulate different envelopes which change shape and effect of the applied current. Threshold modulation of the current's amplitude is used to achieve this goal.

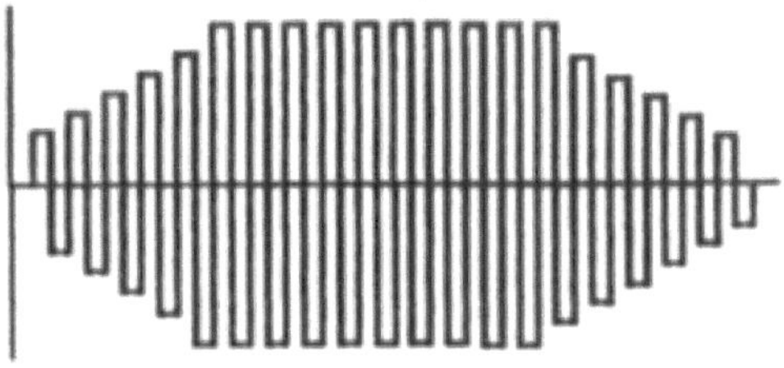

Fig. 43: threshold modulation of Amplitude (trapezoid)

Table 8: The main effects are - according to modulation frequency:

Impulses/minute	Effect
4-6	direct raise of the muscle tone
15	micro massage und stimulation of lymph flow with positive impact on lymph circulation (drainage of the tissues)
30	strong raise of muscle tonicity
60	tensioning and de-tensioning muscle tissue (muscular agitation/shaking)
100	spasmolysis, detonisation of tensed muscles

The threshold amplitude modulation can be modulated from 2-100 oscillations per minute choosing a rectangular or trapezoid shape of the envelope. The modulation depth can be varied from 0 to 75% (but even in modulations below 25% the carrier wave signal i

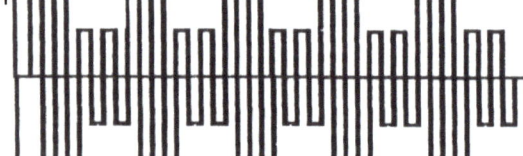

Fig. 44: rectangular amplitude modulation

Table 9: The effects vary depending on the frequency of the envelope (low frequency band):

frequency [Hz]	Therapeutic Effect
100	pain relief, similar to TENS, inhibition of sympathetic nerve system, dilatation of blood vessels, weakening of muscular contraction
50-70	stronger contractions of fast-twitch fibres, slight pain relief
50	stronger contractions of fast- and slow-twitch fibres (superposition), electrical tetanisation of the muscles
20-40	strong but incomplete muscular contractions, slow-twitch fibres, stimulation of parasympathetic nerve system, dilatation of vessels
5-10	tonisation (constriction) of blood vessels, stimulation of the sympathetic nerve system

When „confectioning" the needed form of modulation the frequency from the LFC band is responsible for the current's effect, the MFC is a sort of transport device (carrier wave) that enables the signal to affect the muscle areas through which the current passes.

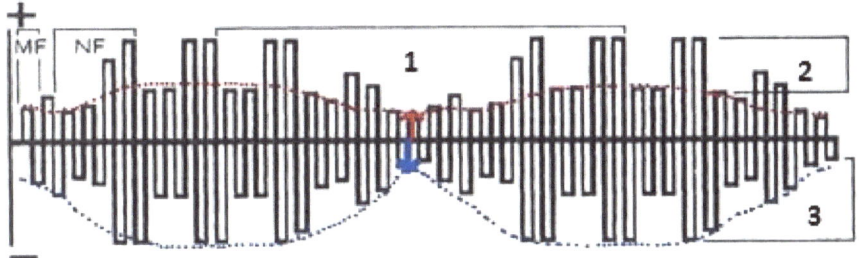

Fig. 45: The MET-Modell
MF: middle frequency (current)
NF: low frequency (current)
1: threshold current
2: intensity of stimulus
3: intensitiy of stimulus thereshold

There is a variety of different effects that can be achieved by using MET:

- Intense muscular stimulation
- Muscular detonisation
- Pain reduction
- Treatment after cerebral apoplectic strokes
- Increasing metabolism to purge cells from toxins and cellular debree

To understand the way MET works one has to be acquainted with three terms often used:

- Gildemeister effect
- Wedensky inhibition
- Senn tonisation.

3.3.1.1 Gildemeister effect:

In comparison with low-frequency current types, there is a difference in the way in which the nerve fibres are depolarized. Due to the higher frequency of the medium-frequency current, not every (alternating current) pulse will result in depolarisation of the nerve fibre. Depolarization of the nerve fibre is the result of the summation principle.

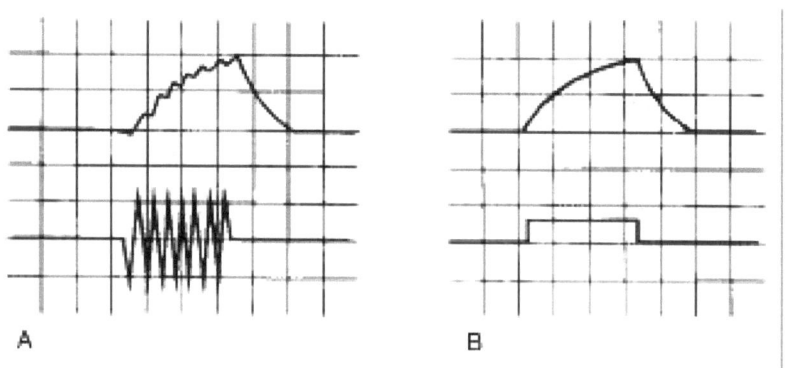

Fig. 46
A. With a medium-frequency current an action potential only arises after a certain number of periods (summation principle).
B. With a direct-current pulse of the same duration an action potential arises at a significantly lower amplitude.

3.3.1.2 Wedensky Inhibition:

Continued stimulation with a medium-frequency alternating current can result in a situation in which the nerve fibre ceases to react to the current (Wedensky inhibition) or the motor end plate becomes fatigued and may fail to transmit the stimulus.

To prevent this, it is necessary to interrupt the current after each depolarization. This can be achieved by rhythmically increasing and decreasing the amplitude (**amplitude modulation***). The Amplitude Modulation Frequency (AMF) determines the frequency of the depolarisation.

The AMF corresponds to the frequencies used in low-frequency electrotherapy.

3.3.1.3 Senn's Tonisation:

This is a result from the above explained phenomena. The slow but continuous local development of the MFC-intensity first causes a lokal contraction in the muscle then spreading continuously in the surrounding muscle tissue and then also slowly fading when the impulse has ended. This distinguishes MFT from LFC or simple MFC stimulation currents.

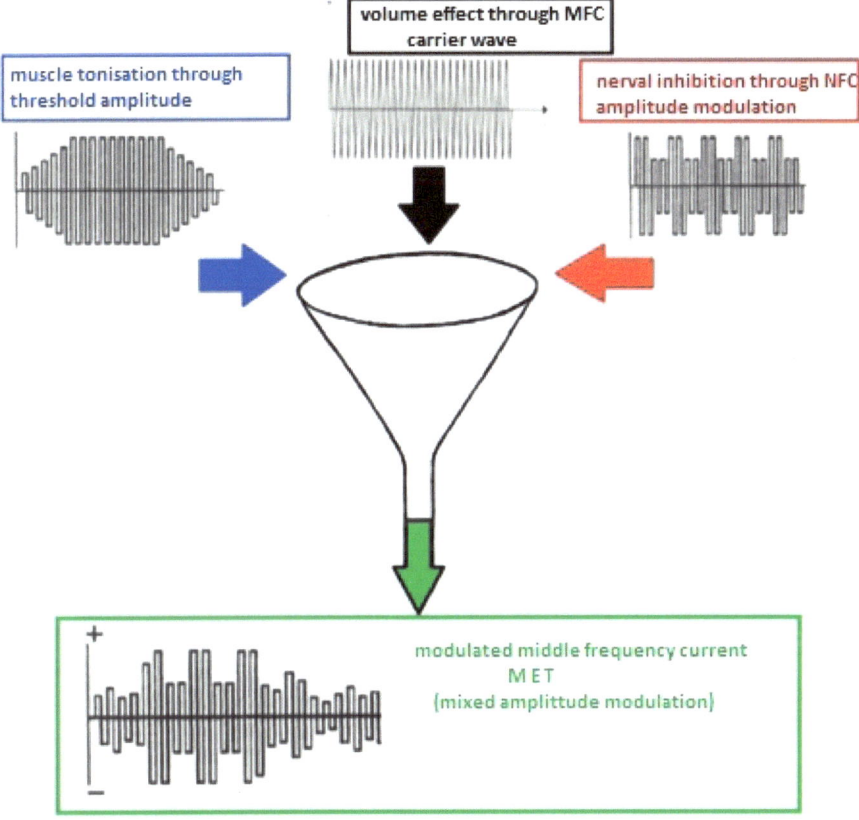

Fig. 47: MET components

Chapter 4: Training of the female Pelvic Floor using MET (EEMA)

4.1 Introduction

The purpose of the training is to build up muscle mass and to prove the patient's perception of the pelvic floor and it's activity which is different from either conventional physiotherapy or LFC intracavital electrotherapy by some points:
- Patients need an experienced therapist who can do the work-out with one (up to two) patient's at a time
- Patients need a whole-body suit, the therapist positions the independent electrodes at the right places
- Programming of the device and regulation of the current is in the hands of the therapist
- There is a basic posture for exercising and different gymnastic exercises depending of what goals have to be achieved, which parts of the musculature have to be trained
- Training the perception of the pelvic floor comes first
- Inner and outer musculature can be trained according to needs
- Additional information on pelvic floor function and disorders should be included in the training

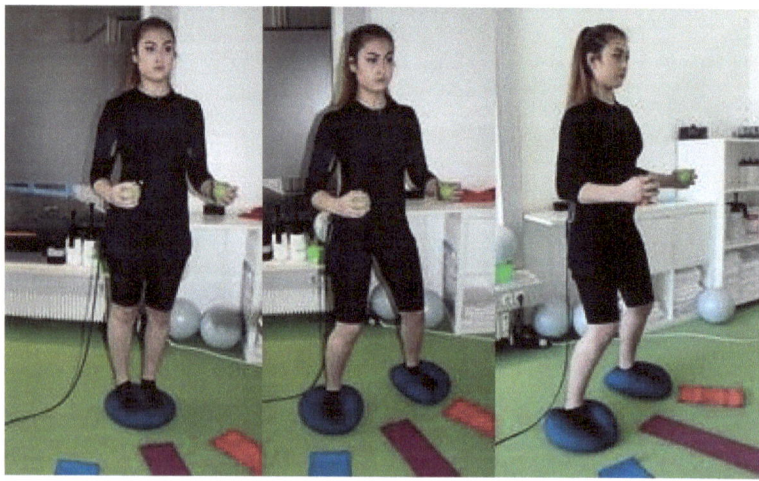

Fig. 48: EEMA-Training

4.2 Glossary

MFC Carrier Wave
A zero line symmetric MFC with steep flanks and mostly a 2-kHz frequency carrying the LF signal that is modulated onto the carrier wave into the tissue but also having effects of its own in the tissue

LFC part of MFT
The low frequency part of the signal sent into the muscle tissue causes a nerve fibre reaction (depolarisation) on a one impulse one action potential basis using the Na^+/K^+-exchange system of the nerve fibre stimulating sensory or motoneurons.

Modulations depth
Its an indicator for the effect of the applied current to the cell membrane and cell itself. It's the percentage of amplitude measuring from the signals peak to the lowest point (remembering that the signal never returns to the zero-line).

Volume effect of MET
There is a homogeneity of flowing current in the tissue using MET for there are no anodes or cathodes involved in MFT (apolarity of MFT).

Index
Amount of current that is working in the patient's body, a relative figure taking sex, age, weight and body height into account). The underwear the patient puts on during exercises reduce the index by approximately 20%.

4.3 Contraindications

There are contraindications for MFT-(EEMA)treatment:

- Electronic implants (pacemaker, pumps, others)
- Arrhythmia
- Cardiac conditions (coronary arteriosclerosis, angina pectoris, myocardial diseases, other vascular problems)
- Pregnancy
- Epilepsy and other convulsive conditions
- Dermatosis (in the areas of electrode positions)
- Thrombosis, phlebitis, arteriosclerosis, peripheral arterial occlusive disease)
- Malignant tumours in the treated area – spare this region
- Breast implants – spare this region
- Acute infectious diseases (respiratory tract, gastro-intestinal tract, acute state of Crohn's disease or ulcerous colitis, acute gall bladder inflammation, gastric ulcers, acute gastritis,...)
- Patient is unfit for exercises.

4.4 Starting Treatment

4.4.1 Preliminaries

Treatment duration: 20 minutes twice a week for initially 18-24 sessions – then evaluation of the therapy's effect

Goals:

- Stabilisation of musculature in general and of the pelvic floor in particular
- Establishing synergies with the abdominal striated muscles and the diaphragm
- Perception of the pelvic floor structures
- Refectory pelvic floor contraction
- Training of power and endurance of contractions
- Activation of the autonomic nervous system
- Working on the bladder's function (storage and voiding).

The different exercises explained, shown and executed are put in a special order including repetitions to meet the patient's individual needs.

We generally start with basic exercises, then introduce variations and repeat the combination of both at least twice to memorise the sequence of exercises and increase their effect. Special adapted breathing techniques and sometimes special exercises are also part of the training.

The first lessons are usually without additional equipment or complex moves so the patient can focus on posture and breathing which in a second step have to be synchronised with the impulses generated by the generator used.

This establishes a relationship between the impulse induced and its effect in the musculature and helps to quickly develop a perception for the pelvic floor muscle structure. This establishes a feeling of control over the musculature.

4.4.2 Placement of Electrodes

For an optimised volume effect of the MFT in the pelvic floor area the thigh-electrodes should be put on firmly (but not too tight) close to the groin.

4.4.3 The use of the chip card

Each pair of electrodes is individually calibrated and the results of this calibration (level of current that can be easily tolerated without causing muscular spasms or cramps) is then stored on the individual's chip card. To train the pelvic floor system there are four pairs of electrodes needed:

- Upper thigh
- Lower back
- Lower abdominal wall
- Buttocks.

5 EEMA-Training - Basics

5.1 Posture
Establish with the patient the term „central line", a straight line connecting the nose, the umbilicus and the pubic symphysis (NUPS-Line) and let the patient focus on the alignment first at rest, then during exercise.

5.2 Breathing
Let the breath flow in and out at all times during the exercises. Breathe with the flow of the current not against it.

5.3 Perception of the musculature
First the patient has to perceive her pelvic floor with the flow of the current. We use the basic posture and simple modifications standing and sitting to achieve the goal of a good perception which is important for further exercises. Then later additional moves or aids (tools) can be added for the exercises

5.4 Perception of the diaphragm
It is important that the patient learns as early as possible that there is a synergism between the work of the pelvic floor, the breathing and the diaphragm. This synergism should be explained, exercised and later practised in real every day life.

5.5 Perception of the pelvic floor
Perception of the musculature and its stabilisation in the lower abdomen and pelvic floor are an essential goal of the MFT. Therefore one part of the exercises is carried out while sitting on a stool or (stabilised) Pezzi® ball. The position (upright upper body; nose, umbilicus and pubic symphysis aligned) has to be controlled (watched and corrected if necessary) by the therapist at all times. Therefore it is best to do the EEMA-Training as an individual training (or train two patients at a time maximum). Legs are equally weighted both feet flat on the floor, the feet in a slightly outward rotated position. Then the current is switched on and with each contraction the patient can perceive her pelvic floor.

5.6 Exercises - Series 1

Goal: Perception of the NUPS-Line and stabilisation of the pelvic floor trough activation of adjacent musculature
a.) adductors
b.) straight abdominal muscles
c.) oblique abdominal muscles

Series 1:

Aids:
Pezzi(R) Ball oder stool
Pelvic floor softball (cf. picture)

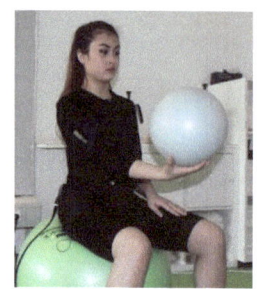

NUPS-Line: • Nose • Umbilicus • Pubic symphysis	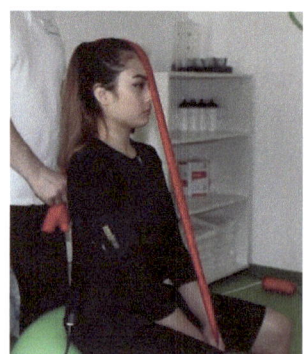
It is important that both ischial tuberosities are symmetrically weighted and that the axis between them forms a right angle with the sternum.	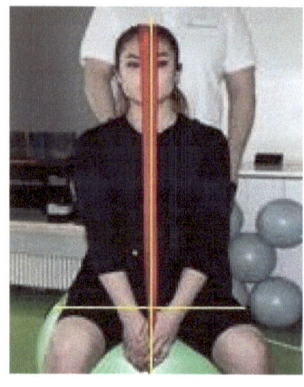

Basic position:
- standing upright
- legs slightly bended
- legs a little bit opened (hip-wide) and
- feet slightly rotated outwards

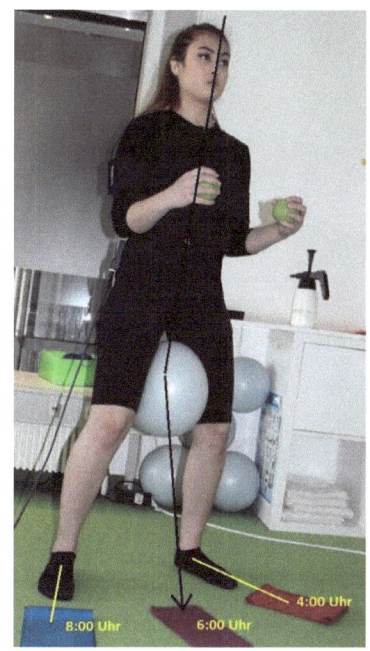

You can see the slightly bended legs, 2/3 of the body's weight rests on the heels, 1/3 on the balls of the feet.

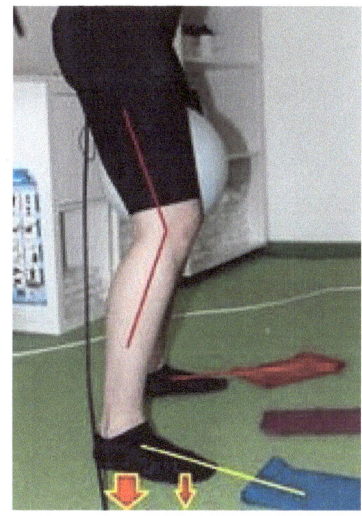

The spinal column is aligned straight and the buttocks are in a slight extension. The glutei muscles are not actively contracted, they will be by the current.	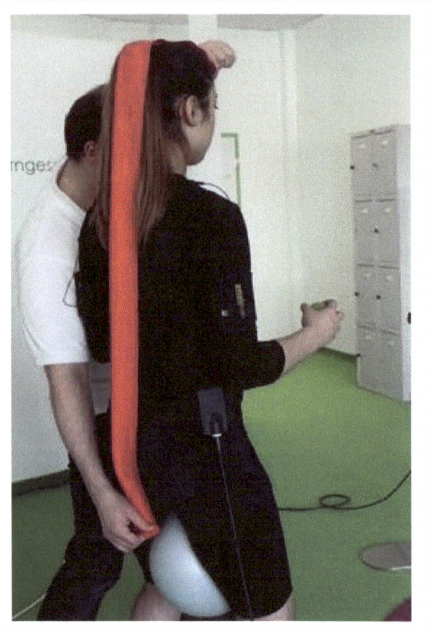
The arms are slightly pressed against the upper body forming a right angle in the elbow joint. Shoulders should be relaxed. Tennis balls are held in both hands facing one another to give the upper body a fixation in the room ("proud chest").	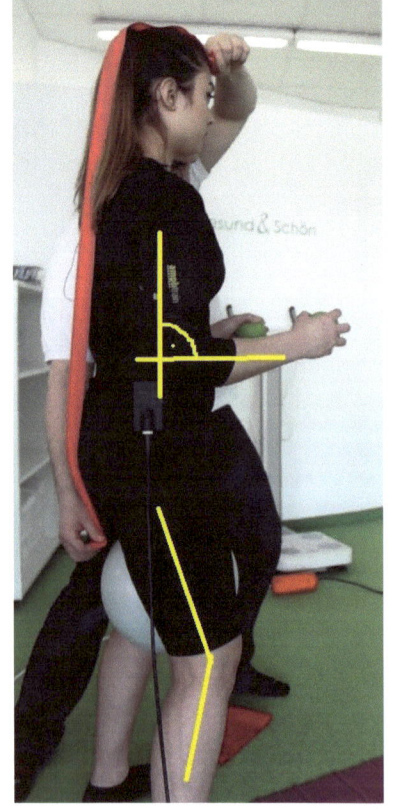

The sternum is also erected which avoids the formation of a (slightly) hollow back with a perceptible tension in the lumbar portion of the spine and the hips. The erection of the sternum comes from the cervical and thoracic spine area with a relaxed neck and shoulder girdle.	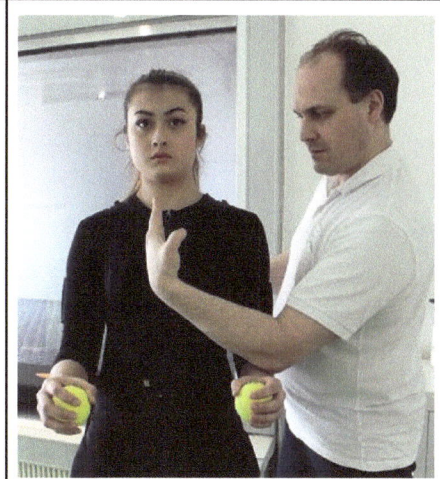
The arms are slightly pressed against the upper body forming a right angle in the elbow joint. Shoulders should be relaxed. Tennis balls are held in both hands facing one another to give the upper body a fixation in the room.	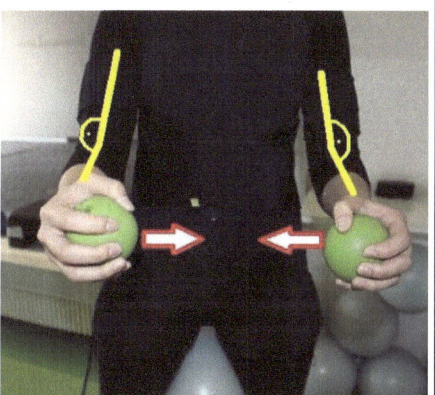
The shoulders should remain relaxed, even a little bit pulled down towards the ground, away from the ears.	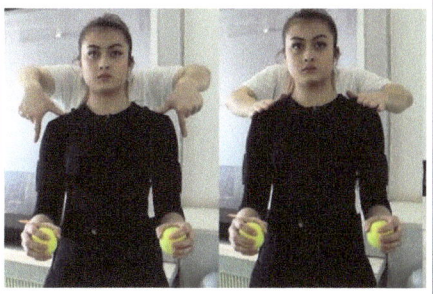

A softball for pelvic floor exercises (25 cm in diameter) is now put between the upper thighs with intense contact to the pubic bone.
The patient will compress the ball when the current impulse increases and the pressure should be kept up for 15-20 seconds, until the impulse decreases again.
The maximum of pressure should be reached in the thighs near to the groins (inguinal region) ["Quadrant of Power"].

The breaks between impulses are "active" - let the current do its effects and only start working into the quadrant of power when the next impulse starts.

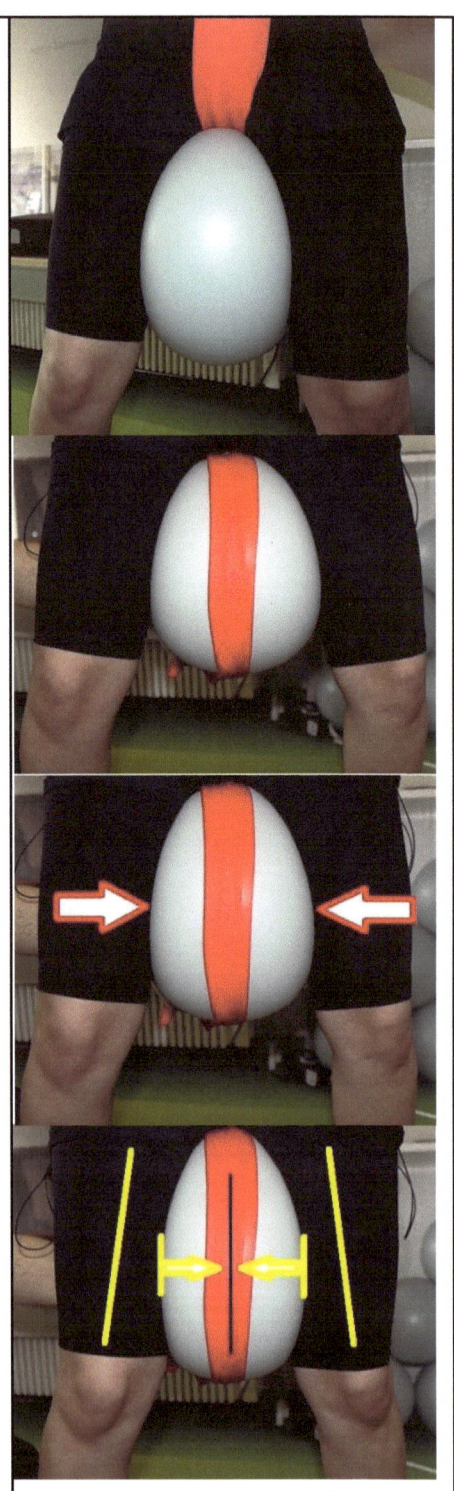

The "Quadrant of Power" is a triangle with a bottom-line between the hipbones the inguinal regions and the adductor muscles (inner side of upper thighs).

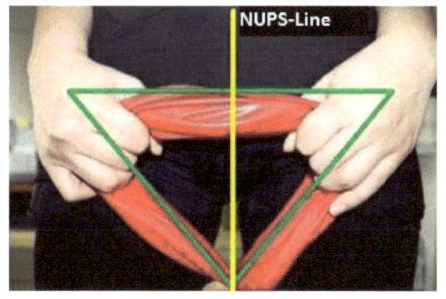

5.7 Series 2 – Exercises sitting down

Aids : Pezzi(R) ball , stool, pelvic floor soft ball, 2 reflex-zone cushions

Patient is sitting on a Pezzi® ball or stool, a pelvic floor soft ball between the upper thighs and both feet placed on a reflex-zone cushion each (they should have a positive impact on the urogenital system).

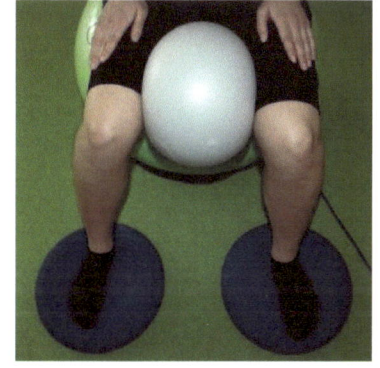

This leads to a involuntary contraction of the adductor muscles, the softball helps the hips to stay stabilised during rest and exercise.

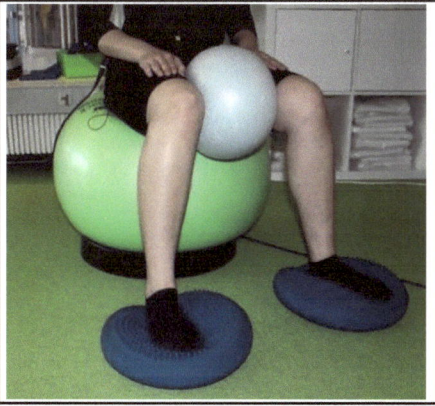

Sitting down the soft ball is in the above described position and slightly fixed with only a little pressure from both thighs. The ball should not go beyond the knee level.

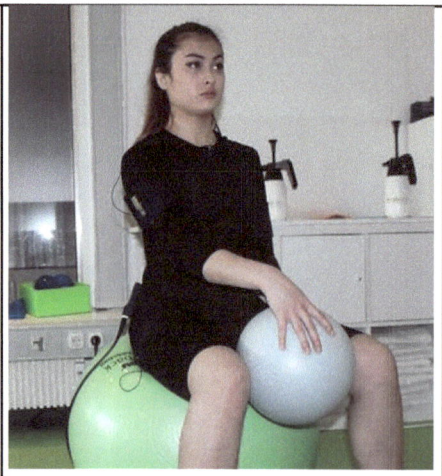

Feet are slightly rotated outwards, the upper body sticks to the above explained posture.

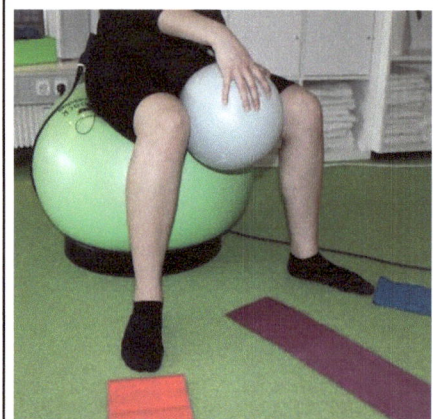

Legs are slightly spread apart, the feet are in firm contact with the ground.

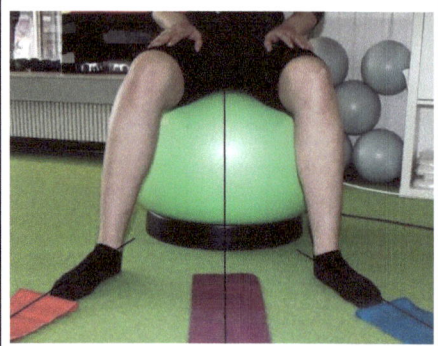

The upper part of the adductor muscles are active. The patient reinforces the impulse when it is increasing, keeps the tension when the impulse has fully developed over the climax' period and then **slowly** relaxes as the impulse decreases again staying relaxed during impulse-free time (active pauses) (avoid sudden abrupt relaxation).

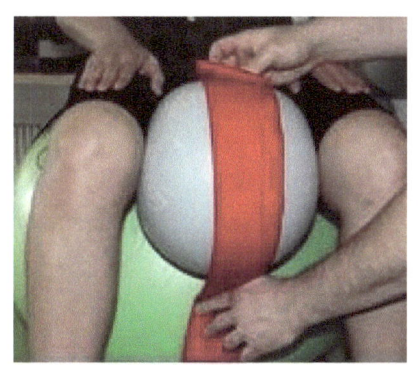

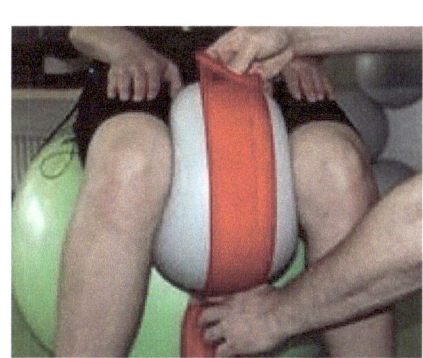

5.8 Series 3: Variations of basic exercises
Variation a:

The Quadrant of Power compresses the softball like bellows when the impulse starts, keeping up approximately 15% of the tension at the end of the impulse during the pause.	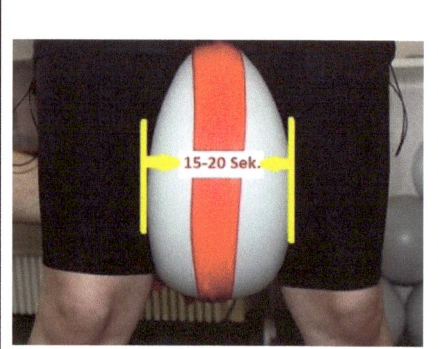
During the pauses the therapist removes the ball and the patient relaxes stepping or walking on the spot or shaking out the legs.	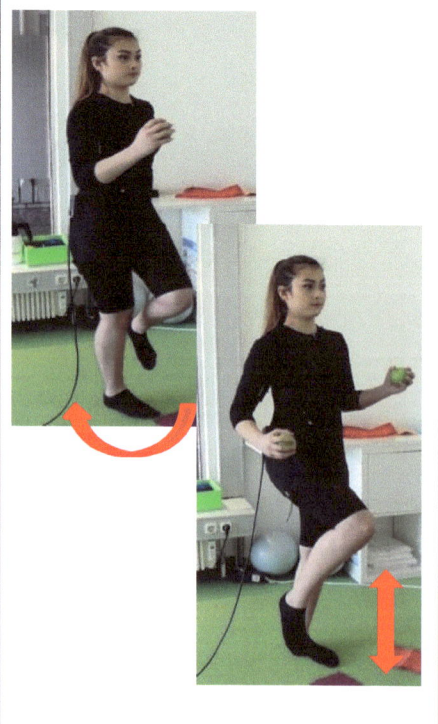

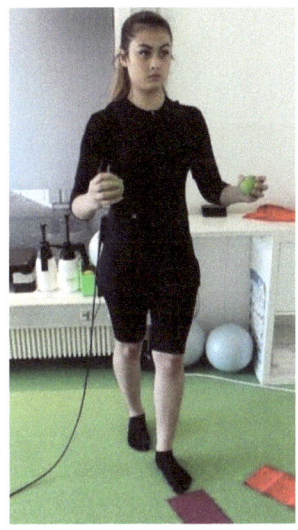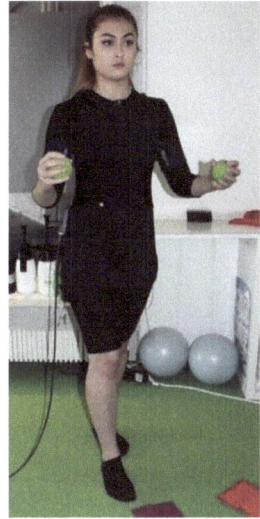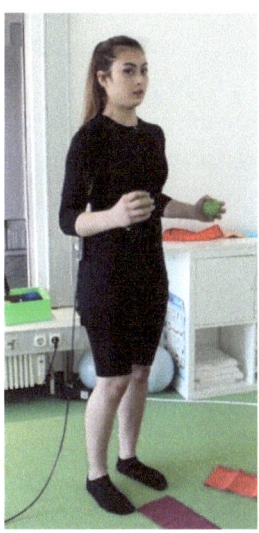

A quick back and forth movement can also be executed in the recess-time.

Variation b:
Switch from compression of the pelvic softball in one period of current flow to pumping movements in the next period. Start when the current starts and end with it when the current starts its decrease. In the impulse-free time make relaxing moves (see above).
Also mind the quality of contraction, rhythm is not important!

Variation c:
-pump the ball up with more air so it becomes harder
-change the ball's diameter (larger)
This means that you need more effort to compress and that is good to build up more musculature.

In this context it is important to mind the basic posture and the upright position. That limits the degree of air you can pump into the ball or the diameter you can choose because the hips should not be pushed apart too far which would cause tension in the lumbar portion of the spine or pelvis. Especially be careful with patients with hip or knee prosthesis.

To close we would like to give the following recommendations:

Breathing: during exercise the patient should calmly in- and exhale

Posture: watch out for NUSP-line at all times.

„Active" Pauses: do not forget to ask the patient to practice an active relaxation during the signal-free periods (shaking of the legs, walking on the spot)

pelvic floor softball: focus on the Quadrant of Power, keep approximately 15% of the pressure on the soft ball during pauses. Knees, buttocks and upper body are not contracting in this particular exercise-setting.

Focus: keep the patient focussed on NUPS-line, Quadrant of Power and the signal to be seen on the display which makes the acting current visible.

Home training: since January 2017 EEMA-generators are available for home-training as well. After having practised EEMA under surveillance of a therapist for a certain period they can be prescribed and the training can be done at home approximately twice a week. In the beginning it is advisable to have someone watch the patient's posture, breathing and the way the exercises are carried out to eliminate mistakes as early as possible.

5.9 General recommendations for the user:

- Do not exercise after meals
- Try to exercise at about the same time each day you perform your training
- Drink approximately 500 ml water/tea before starting the exercises and about the same amount afterwards
- Keep at least 48 hours between the sessions
- Don't overdo work-out and other physical activity on your EEMA-days
- When training on your own watch the DVD more than once and study this manual before starting your exercises
- EEMA is just one puzzle-stone in the conservative treatment of pelvic floor disorders, in many cases it has to be accompanied by other forms of treatment to obtain a good result.

6 Acknowledgements

We thank Leah Lehmann for her patience and endurance during the shooting sessions which enabled us to really show therapists and users the principles of the treatment.

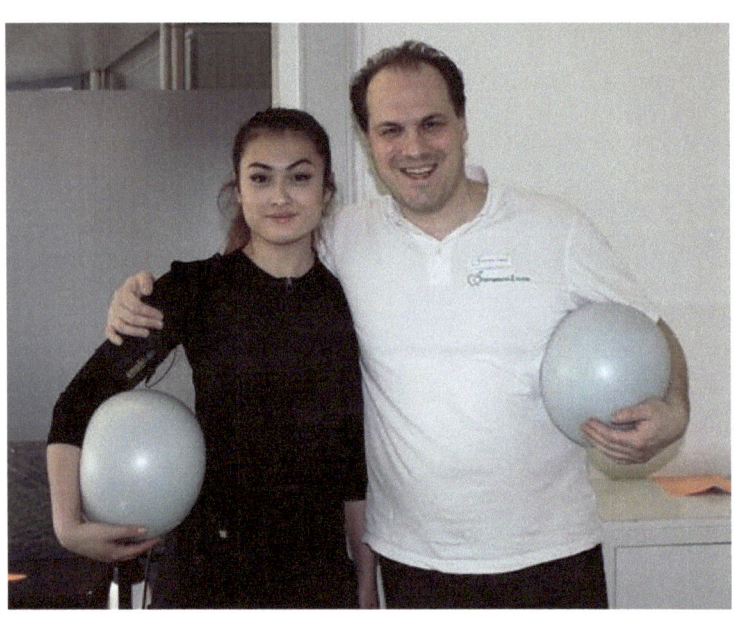

Dr. med. Armin Fischer
Head of Department
St. Josefs-Hospital Rheingau
Eibinger Straße 9
D-65385 Rüdesheim/Rhein
Tel.: +49-6722/490-390
Email:
afischer@joho-rheingau.de
Web:
www.drarminfischer.jimdo.com

Alexander Lehman
Schwarzgasse 2
65191 Wiesbaden
Deutsche Gesellschaft für
Beckenbodengesundheit e.V.
(German Association for Pelvic Floor Health)
Email:
lehmanalexander03@googlemail.com
Web:
https://beckenboden-gesundheit.org

Chapter	Title	Page
1	The Pelvic Floor – structure and function	4
1.1	Anatomy – the bascis	4
1.2	Continence and Integral Theory (IT)	7
1.2.1	Continence and bladder function according to the IT	8
1.3	Diagnostic Algorithm	18
1.3.1	Explenation of Diagnostic Algorithm	20
1.3.1.1	Anterior Zone Defects	20
1.3.1.2	Posterior Zone Defects	22
1.3.1.3	Detrusor Instability (DI)	24
1.4	Stability of the Pelvic Floor System (PFS)	26
1.5	Anterior wall defects	29
1.5.1	Midline defects	30
1.5.2	Lateral defects	31
1.6	Posterior wall defects	33
1.6.1	Rectocele	33
1.6.2	Enterocele	34
2	Basics of Conventional Treatment	35
2.1	Hormones - Oestrogens	35
2.2	PVA-Tampons	36
2.3	Pessary tretment	40
2.3.1	The use of ring-shaped pessaries	41
2.3.2	The use of cubic pessaries	42
2.4	Pelvic floor physiotherapy	44
	Part II	
3.1	Conventional Electrophjysiotherapy	51
3.2	Biofeedback Therapy	52
3.3	EEMA Treatment	53
3.3.1	Modulated middle frequency electrotherapy (MFT, EEMA)	55
3.3.1.1	Gildemeister Effect	58
3.3.1.2	Wedensky Inhibition	58
3.3.1.3	Senn's Tonisation	59
4	Training of the pelvic floor with MET	60
4.1	Introduction	60

Chapter	Title	Page
4.2	Glossary	61
4.3	Contraindications	62
4.4	Starting treatment	63
4.4.1	Preliminaries	63
4.4.2	Placement of electrodes	64
4.4.3	Use of chip card	64
5	EEMA-Training – Basics	65
5.1	Posture	65
5.2	Breathing	65
5.3	Perception of musculature	65
5.4	Perception of the diaphragm	65
5.5	Perception of the pelvic floor	65
5.6	Exercises – Series 1	66
5.7	Exercises – Series 2	71
5.8	Exercises – Series 3	74
5.9	General recommandations for the user	77
6	Aknowledgements	78

www.ingramcontent.com/pod-product-compliance
Lightning Source LLC
Chambersburg PA
CBHW040225220526
45473CB00001B/118